Pocket Guideline of
Diabetic Foot
For Professionals

AF070620

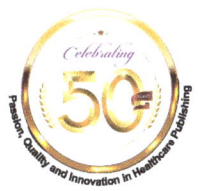

Pocket Guideline of
Diabetic Foot
For Professionals

Second Edition

Editors

Zulfiqarali G Abbas MBBS DTM&H (UK) MMed FRCP (Glasg)
Consultant Physician, Endocrinologist, and Diabetologist
Founder and Chairman, Pan-African Diabetic Foot Study Group
Vice-President, D-Foot International
Executive Member of Infection Committee
International Working Group on the Diabetic Foot (IWGDF)
Department of Internal Medicine, Abbas Medical Centre
Muhimbili University of Health and Allied Sciences
Dar es Salaam, Tanzania

Arun Bal MS PhD
Consultant Diabetic Foot Surgeon
Founder and President, Diabetic Foot Society of India
Department of Diabetic Foot Surgery
Raheja Hospital, Hinduja Hospital, Mumbai, Maharashtra, India
Visiting Professor
Amrita Institute of Medical Sciences, Kochi, Kerala, India

Forewords

Andrew JM Boulton
Kristien Van Acker

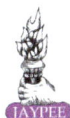

JAYPEE BROTHERS MEDICAL PUBLISHERS
The Health Sciences Publisher
New Delhi | London | Panama

Jaypee Brothers Medical Publishers (P) Ltd

Headquarters
Jaypee Brothers Medical Publishers (P) Ltd
4838/24, Ansari Road, Daryaganj
New Delhi 110 002, India
Phone: +91-11-43574357
Fax: +91-11-43574314
Email: jaypee@jaypeebrothers.com

Overseas Offices

J.P. Medical Ltd
83 Victoria Street, London
SW1H 0HW (UK)
Phone: +44 20 3170 8910
Fax: +44 (0)20 3008 6180
Email: info@jpmedpub.com

Jaypee-Highlights Medical Publishers Inc
City of Knowledge, Bld. 235, 2nd Floor, Clayton
Panama City, Panama
Phone: +1 507-301-0496
Fax: +1 507-301-0499
Email: cservice@jphmedical.com

Jaypee Brothers Medical Publishers (P) Ltd
Bhotahity, Kathmandu, Nepal
Phone: +977-9741283608
Email: kathmandu@jaypeebrothers.com

Website: www.jaypeebrothers.com
Website: www.jaypeedigital.com

© 2019, Jaypee Brothers Medical Publishers

The views and opinions expressed in this book are solely those of the original contributor(s)/author(s) and do not necessarily represent those of editor(s) of the book.

All rights reserved. No part of this publication may be reproduced, stored or transmitted in any form or by any means, electronic, mechanical, photocopying, recording or otherwise, without the prior permission in writing of the publishers.

All brand names and product names used in this book are trade names, service marks, trademarks or registered trademarks of their respective owners. The publisher is not associated with any product or vendor mentioned in this book.

Medical knowledge and practice change constantly. This book is designed to provide accurate, authoritative information about the subject matter in question. However, readers are advised to check the most current information available on procedures included and check information from the manufacturer of each product to be administered, to verify the recommended dose, formula, method and duration of administration, adverse effects and contraindications. It is the responsibility of the practitioner to take all appropriate safety precautions. Neither the publisher nor the author(s)/editor(s) assume any liability for any injury and/or damage to persons or property arising from or related to use of material in this book.

This book is sold on the understanding that the publisher is not engaged in providing professional medical services. If such advice or services are required, the services of a competent medical professional should be sought.

Every effort has been made where necessary to contact holders of copyright to obtain permission to reproduce copyright material. If any have been inadvertently overlooked, the publisher will be pleased to make the necessary arrangements at the first opportunity. The **CD/DVD-ROM** (if any) provided in the sealed envelope with this book is complimentary and free of cost. **Not meant for sale.**

Inquiries for bulk sales may be solicited at: jaypee@jaypeebrothers.com

Pocket Guideline of Diabetic Foot: For Professionals / Zulfiqarali G Abbas, Arun Bal

First Edition: 2014
Second Edition: 2019
ISBN: 978-93-5270-313-5

Contributors

EDITORS

Zulfiqarali G Abbas MBBS DTM&H (UK) MMed FRCP (Glasg)
Consultant Physician, Endocrinologist, and Diabetologist
Founder and Chairman, Pan-African Diabetic Foot Study Group
Vice-President, D-Foot International
Executive Member of Infection Committee
International Working Group on the Diabetic Foot (IWGDF)
Department of Internal Medicine, Abbas Medical Centre
Muhimbili University of Health and Allied Sciences
Dar es Salaam, Tanzania

Arun Bal MS PhD
Consultant Diabetic Foot Surgeon
Founder and President, Diabetic Foot Society of India
Department of Diabetic Foot Surgery
Raheja Hospital, Hinduja Hospital, Mumbai, Maharashtra, India
Visiting Professor
Amrita Institute of Medical Sciences, Kochi, Kerala, India

CONTRIBUTING AUTHORS

Lynne Tudhope MBChB MMED BA
Department of Vascular Surgery and Endovascular Surgery
Head, Multidisciplinary Diabetic Foot Clinic
Wilgers Hospital
Pretoria, South Africa

Hanan Gawish PhD MD
Professor of Diabetes and Endocrinology
Department of Internal Medicine
Mansoura University
Mansoura, Egypt

Mamdouh Radwan El-Nahas MD
Professor of Endocrinology and Diabetes
Head, Department of Internal Medicine
Port Said University
Port Said, Egypt

Howard E Alexander Msc Med (Wits)
Podiatrist in Private Practice
Part-time Lecturer, Sport Scientist
Department of Podiatry
University of Johannesburg, University of Witwatersrand
Johannesburg, South Africa

Liezl Naude BCur MCur IIWCC
Wound Management Specialist
Consultant, Wound Care
Eloquent Health and Wellness
Pretoria, Gauteng, South Africa

Foreword

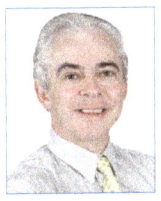

Andrew JM Boulton MD DSc (Hon) FACP FICP FRCP
Professor of Medicine, University of Manchester, Manchester, UK
Visiting Professor, University of Miami, Miami, FL, USA
Consultant Physician, Manchester Royal Infirmary, Manchester, UK
Past-President, European Association for the Study of Diabetes
President, Worldwide Initiative for Diabetes Education
Chair, EURADIA (Alliance for European Diabetes Research)
President-Elect (2018–19), International Diabetes Federation

It is a pleasure to write the foreword for the second edition of what has proven to be a most popular and successful pocket booklet on Diabetic Foot Disease.

Diabetic foot complications are responsible for much morbidity and even mortality across the world and the African continent is no exception to this rule. Indeed, the majority of foot lesions in this part of the world occur secondary to sensory loss as a consequence of diabetic peripheral neuropathy. Many patients have, therefore, lost "the gift of pain" and are at risk of developing foot lesions as a consequence of insensitivity together with trauma which may simply be caused by barefoot walking. Although peripheral arterial disease is increasing in its prevalence in this continent, it is still much less prevalent than in other parts of the world particularly Western countries. Thus, most foot problems should be eminently preventable and as stated in this pocket book, identification of the high risk foot is easily achieved by a quick foot exam and does not require any expensive equipment. Indeed, simple tools such as a monofilament, a tuning fork, and so on are all that is needed together with a careful inspection of the foot.

Dr Abbas has amassed an excellent team of contributors to this remarkable pocket book but in this second edition has added a well-known surgeon on the diabetic foot, Dr Arun Bal, who is not only known in India, but also internationally for his excellent work. The team is to be congratulated for producing such a beautifully illustrated and simple pocket book that should be of use to all health care practitioners looking after patients with diabetes. The emphasis on prevention and the establishment of even a minimal diabetic foot care team is so important and is given prominence throughout this excellent monograph. The addition of surgery to this text is entirely appropriate and of course the diabetic foot surgeon is a vital member of the diabetic foot care team. It is, therefore, my hope that this pocket book will update the readership on this all too common problem and give very simple and practical approaches to the prevention and medical and surgical treatment of this very serious complication of diabetes.

Foreword

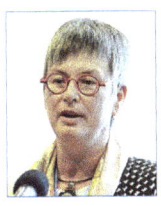

Kristien Van Acker MD PhD
Consultant Physician, Diabetes and Endocrinology
President, D-Foot International (Former Implementation Group of
International Working Group of Diabetic Foot)
Department of Internal Medicine, Diabetology, and Endocrinology
Centre Santé des Fagnes
Chimay, Belgium

The prevalence of diabetes throughout the world is increasing. In 2017, global prevalence of diabetes was estimated at 424.9 million and this figure is predicted to reach 628.6 million by 2045. Of which 80% live in low- and middle-income countries.

Globally, up to 70% of all leg amputations happen to people with diabetes. Every 20 seconds a lower limb is lost to diabetes somewhere in the world. The fact that the prevalence of diabetes increases so rapidly there is the need for appropriate preventive and management strategies, especially education.

The spread of best practice of care and research findings is essential in improving the quality of life of people with diabetes and suffering from complications like the diabetic foot syndrome.

I like to remember that the first Step-by-Step program was launched in 2003 in Africa of which editor Dr Zulfiqarali G Abbas was one of the founding fathers and has already being successfully executed in many countries with a huge outcome of many interdisciplinary diabetic foot clinics. This was the real breakthrough for reduction in amputations in the developing countries. Those programs are the basis of many others in developing countries, where diabetic foot had almost no attention. Dr Zulfiqarali G Abbas has shown for the first time that the "Step-by-Step" project in his country has significantly reduced the number of amputations by 50%. This widely recognized success of these programs has certainly played an important role in the growing awareness of this process.

Step by step leads to formation of the train the trainer program which has now being successfully executed in four regions across the globe. First was held in Brazil followed by Carrabin, Europe, and Western Pacific.

I am extremely pleased and honored to be part of this second edition of the pocket diabetic foot guidelines from Africa and Asia. It is first of its kind covering both the medical and surgical aspects on the diabetic foot.

The publication of this important 2nd edition of the *Pocket Guideline of Diabetic Foot* on diabetic foot care will eliminate misconceptions related to the medical and surgical aspects of the treatment of the diabetic limbs. It will definitely improve the management and prevention of the diabetic foot. I hope this booklet will find its way to many health care workers in the field, which will contribute to less suffering of the patient and will lead to a reduction of the still unacceptable high number of limb amputation.

As the President of the D-Foot International Implementation Group of Internal Working Group on Diabetic Foot, I would like to congratulate the chairman of the Pan-African Diabetic Foot Study group Dr Zulfiqarali G Abbas and his team and Chairman of Diabetic Foot Society of India Dr Arun Bal, and all those involved in bringing this pocket booklet. We applaud their hard work in producing such an impressive and interesting book on diabetic foot.

Preface to the Second Edition

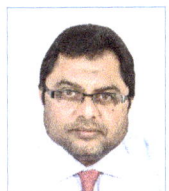

Zulfiqarali G Abbas
MBBS DTM&H (UK) MMed FRCP (Glasg)

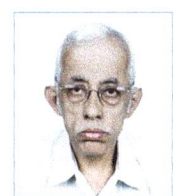

Arun Bal
MS PhD

Diabetes is reaching epidemic proportions across the globe. It is one of the few diseases that affects multiple organ systems. Some of the most feared complications of diabetes for those people who have the misfortune to develop it are lower limb disease, foot ulceration, infection, amputation, and ultimately death.

Until recently, diabetic foot disease has been a relatively neglected complication of diabetes, but slowly things are changing. Patients, health care workers and policy makers have started to realize the quite staggering burden of foot disease for individuals and society. Evidence of this may be seen in the ever increasing numbers of scientific publications on the diabetic foot disease.

Diabetes is a truly multi-organ disease, it requires input from a variety of health care specialists, none of whom should be expected to manage these complications in isolation. Indeed, for many specialists, diabetes related foot disease represents the most challenging aspects of their individual specialty.

If lower limbs and specially foot complications are managed in a timely and expert fashion, ulcers will be healed, limbs preserved, and lives saved. Delayed or poor management, including failure to use evidence based therapies, will result in ulcers that fail to heal, leading to amputations and death.

Education remains the basic tenet for the prevention of complications among persons with diabetes. More than that, education remains the key component of good self-care that in many ways remains a fundamental human right and influence the quality of life of any preventive program—it should be simple and repetitive and targeted at health care providers as well as patients themselves, relatives, and friends.

This second edition of the pocket guideline is a useful tool for clinical practice aimed at managing the diabetic foot; it focuses on the key aspects of prevention and education through initiatives based on sharing knowledge. In this second edition of the pocket guideline, we have added surgical aspects of diabetic foot.

Together with the initiative from D-Foot International implementation section of International Working Group on Diabetic Foot, Pan-African Diabetic Foot Study Group, and Diabetic Foot Society of India, our hope is that this guideline will serve as a useful ancillary tool by providing essential information aimed at improving diabetic foot care.

This second edition of *Pocket Guideline of Diabetic Foot* care provides a broad sweep of current knowledge in the field of medical and surgical aspects of the diabetic foot complications. It is our hope that you will find this second edition informative and rewarding and we look forward to future third edition in which further evidence based data and progress aimed at improving patient outcome can be reported.

Preface to the First Edition

At present, the number of amputations resulting from diabetic foot complications remains unacceptably high. Moreover, foot ulcer generally precede most of these diabetes-associated amputations. The most important risk factor for acquiring a diabetic ulcer in out part of the world is peripheral neuropathy, followed by peripheral arterial disease and mixed pathology (i.e., presence of both neuropathy and peripheral arterial disease). Compounding the problem is the increasing morbidity and mortality associated with infection of the unlcers themselves, underlying soft tissues, and bone. Infection at any of these anatomic sites can progress to systemic infection and ultimately death.

Published data suggests that rates of lower limb amputation can be reduced by as much as 85% through implementation of a multi-disciplinary approach to a foot ulcer management that include close monitoring of patients, and education of persons with diabetes as well as the health care provider themselves. Education remains the basic tenet for the prevention of complications among persons with diabetes. More than that education remains the key component of good self-care that in many ways remains a fundamental human right in that it can influence the quality of life of a person or even make a difference between life and death. Thus, education of patients and health care workers should be an integral part of any prevention program. It should be simple and repetitive and targeted at health care providers (i.e., doctors, nurses, and ancillary staff) as well as patients themselves, relatives, and friends. This pocket guideline is a useful tool for clinical practice aimed at managing the diabetic foot; it focuses on the key aspects of prevention and education through initiatives based on sharing of knowledge.

Together with the initiative from the International Working Group on Diabetic Foot and the Pan-African Diabetic Foot Study Group, my hope is that this guideline will serve as a useful ancillary tool by providing essential information aimed at improving diabetic foot care.

This edition of *Pocket Guideline of Diabetic Foot* care provides a broad sweep of current knowledge in the field of diabetic foot complications. It is my hope that you will find this first edition informative and rewarding and I look forward to a future second edition in which further evidence-based data and progress aimed at improving patient outcomes can be reported.

Zulfiqarali G Abbas

Acknowledgments

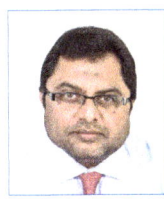

Zulfiqarali G Abbas
MBBS DTM&H (UK) MMed FRCP (Glasg)

The words "thank you" do not truly reflect my immense sense of gratitude as I publish this pocket booklet on the diabetic foot. This task would have hardly been possible without the help of so many people.

To start with, I am very much grateful to Almighty God for giving me the opportunity, strength, and fortitude to enable change and improvement of outcomes among persons with diabetic foot complications in under-privileged countries. Next, I should like to thank my parents, without whose love, support, and encouragement I would never have accomplished my current academic and professional standing or been able to reach and help the many disadvantaged patients with diabetes.

It is my great pleasure to thank eminent experts from across the globe, who readily accepted my invitation and in timely fashion contributed to this pocket booklet on diabetic foot issues. Here, I should like to take the opportunity to thank the following individuals for providing me with full support: Professor Andrew JM Boulton, President, Worldwide Initiative for Diabetes Education, President-Elect, International Diabetes Federation, Past-President of European Association for the Study of Diabetes and Dr Kristien Van Acker, President of D-Foot International (former International Working Group on the Diabetic Foot-IWGDF – implementation group).

I should also like to thank the entire executive board members of the Pan-African Diabetic Foot Study Group, the team of the Step-by-Step Diabetic Foot project and Train the Foot Trainer project, academic and research colleagues, and the various experts in the field of diabetic foot complications for their continued support and contributions to this book, which is aimed at improving care for people with diabetes in Africa and other economically less-developed countries. In this second edition of the *Pocket Guideline of Diabetic Foot*, I would like to thank Dr Arun Bal for his great contribution on the section of surgical aspects of diabetic foot. I should also like to thank in particularly my research and academic colleagues—Professor Lennox K Archibald and Professor Janet Lutale—for being very supportive and for collaborating with me in the conduct of various clinical, epidemiologic, and microbiologic studies relevant to better understanding of the diabetic foot in underprivileged settings.

Over the past two and half decades, I have learnt a lot from my patients who are actually open textbooks. I should like to thank them collectively for giving me the opportunity to treat them and to learn from them.

The list of acknowledgments would be incomplete without a thought or mention of family. As always, I should like to highlight the debt I owe to members of my own family—my wife and children—for their patience, quiet support, and understanding during the inevitable periods when work on the manuscript or related travel intruded on our family life.

Contents

Section 1: Medical Aspect of Diabetic Foot

1. Diabetes Mellitus—A Clinical Challenge 3
2. Top Ten Countries for Number of Adults with Diabetes 4
3. Epidemiology of the Diabetic Foot 5
4. Economical Burden of the Diabetic Foot Ulcer 6
5. Pathway to Diabetic Foot Ulcer 7
6. Factors Associated with Foot Ulcer 8
7. Pathophysiology of Foot Ulceration 9
8. Diabetic Peripheral Neuropathy 10
9. Types of Peripheral Neuropathy 11
10. Tests for Peripheral Neuropathy 12
11. Vibration Test 13
12. Biothesiometer or Neuro-esthesiometer 14
13. Other Tests for Peripheral Neuropathy 15
14. Neuropad (Autonomic Test) 16
15. Neuro-osteoarthropathy (Charcot Foot) 17
16. Indications for a Neurological Referral in Patients with Suspected Diabetic Sensorimotor Neuropathy 18
17. Oral Symptomatic Therapies in Painful Diabetic Neuropathy 19
18. Peripheral Arterial Diseases 20
19. Stages of Peripheral Arterial Disease 21
20. Chronic Critical Ischemia 22
21. Classification of Peripheral Arterial Disease 23

22.	Interpretation of the Ankle-brachial Index	24
23.	Computed Tomography Scan Angiogram of Lower Limbs	25
24.	Transcutaneous Oxygen Monitor	26
25.	Clinical Symptoms of Neuropathic and Ischemic Foot Ulcers	27
26.	Neuroischemic Diabetic Foot (Mixed)	29
27.	Diabetic Foot Infections	30
28.	Risk Factors for Infection	31
29.	Three Most Important Clinical Categories of Infections	32
30.	Cellulitis	33
31.	Deep Soft Tissue Infection	34
32.	Chronic Osteomyelitis	35
33.	Criteria for Diagnosis of Osteomyelitis	36
34.	Typical Features of Diabetic Foot Osteomyelitis on Plain X-rays	37
35.	Classification and Severity of Infection	38
36.	Indications of Worsening Infection	39
37.	Characteristics Suggesting a More Serious Diabetic Foot Infection and Potential Indications for Hospitalization	40
38.	Factors that May Influence Choices of Antibiotics Therapy for Diabetic Foot Infections (Specific Agents, Route of Administration, Duration of Therapy)	42
39.	Factors Potentially Favoring Selecting Either Primarily Antibiotics or Surgical Resection for Diabetic Foot Osteomyelitis	43
40.	Antibiotic Regimens for Mild, Moderate, and Severe Diabetic Foot Infections	44

41.	Duration of Treatment for Infected Diabetic Foot	46
42.	Wagner Classification	48
43.	PEDIS Classification	49
44.	The University of Texas Classification	51
45.	SINDBAD Classification	52
46.	Lower Extremity Threatened Limb Classification System	53
47.	Ischemia: Clinical Category	54
48.	Foot Infection: Clinical Category	55
49.	Simple Staging of the Diabetic Foot	56
50.	Consider the Whole Patient and not the Hole in the Patient to Ensure Effective Care of the Foot Ulcer	58
51.	Foot Examination	59
52.	Ulcer Assessment	60
53.	Wound Bed	61
54.	Examination of Edge, Wall, and Base	62
55.	A Summary of the Management of Diabetic Foot Ulcer	63
56.	Local Wound Treatment	65
57.	Role of Debridement in Ulcer Management	66
58.	Debridement Methods and Its Characteristics	67
59.	Summary of Indications for Different Dressings/Devices	68
60.	Ulcer Healing	69
61.	Surgical Intervention in Severe Cases where Abnormal Pressure Distribution is Causing Persistent and Nonresolvable Ulceration	70
62.	Biomechanics Factors and Footwear	71

63.	Plantar Pressure Reduction	72
64.	Footwear and Offloading for the Diabetic Foot: An Evidence-based Guideline	73
65.	General Guide to Footwear Based on Risk Status	74
66.	Examination of the Insensate Diabetic Foot	75
67.	The Diabetic Foot Ulcers: Outcome and Management	76
68.	Global Burden of Limb Amputation	77
69.	Preventing Diabetic Foot Amputation	78
70.	Nonulcerative Pathology of Ulcers	79
71.	Social Factors of the Diabetic Foot	81
72.	Time is Tissue in the Diabetic Foot	82
73.	Pathway to Clinical Care for Diabetic Foot Ulcer	83
74.	Risk Categorization System	84
75.	How to Prevent Foot Problems	85
76.	Ulcer Prevention	86
77.	Training of Health Care Workers	87
78.	The Step-by-Step Diabetic Foot Project	88
79.	Train the Foot Trainer Project	89
80.	Organization of Foot Care	90
81.	The Minimal Foot Clinic Model	91
82.	Pathway of Refer for Foot Care	92
83.	Tropical Diabetic Hand Syndrome	93
84.	Algorithm for Management of Tropical Diabetic Hand Syndrome	94
85.	Issues—Particular Importance in Developing Countries	95

Section 2: Surgical Aspect of Diabetic Foot

86.	Diabetes Mellitus—Surgical Challenge	99
87.	Team Approach	100
88.	Foot Salvage Surgery	101
89.	Neuropathy and Surgery	102
90.	Charcot Foot	103
91.	Imaging in Charcot Foot	105
92.	Indication for Surgical Treatment	106
93.	Surgical Treatment for Charcot Foot	107
94.	Choice of Surgical Procedures	108
95.	Healing Time in Surgical Treatment of Charcot Foot	109
96.	Complication of Surgical Treatment	110
97.	Peripheral Arterial Disease and Surgery	111
98.	How Peripheral Arterial Disease is Different in Diabetes than Nondiabetic Patients	112
99.	Peripheral Arterial Disease, Transcutaneous Oxygen Pressure, and Surgery	113
100.	Imaging Modalities	114
101.	Selection of Type of Imaging	115
102.	When and How to Treat Foot Gangrene When Revascularization is not Feasible	116
103.	Selection of Type of Revascularization	117
104.	Steps to Prevent Acute Kidney Injury in a Susceptible Patient	118
105.	Use of Non-iodine Based Contrast	119

106.	Post-revascularization Treatment	121
107.	Schedule for Antibiotics is as Follows	122
108.	Post-revascularization Prevention	123
109.	Necrotizing Fasciitis	124
110.	Osteomyelitis	128
111.	The Conservative Treatment of Osteomyelitis	129
112.	Debridement in Patients with Infection and Vasculopathy	130
113.	Conservative Management of Localized Gangrene	131
114.	Factors That Influence Wound Closure Procedure	132
115.	Factors That Retard Healing	133
116.	Commonly Used Procedures within Each Surgical Category	134
117.	Different Types of Dressing	138
118.	Acute Wound Flowchart	139
119.	Chronic Wound Flowchart	140
120.	Skin Grafting in Diabetic Foot	142
121.	Advantages of Split Thickness Skin Graft	143
122.	Local/Regional Anesthesia for Diabetic Foot Surgery	145
123.	Total Contact Cast for Diabetic Foot Patients	151
124.	Advantages of Contact Casting in Diabetic Foot Ulcers	152
125.	Contraindication for Total Contact Casting in Diabetic Foot Ulcers	153
126.	Why Diabetes Patients Gets Bilateral Pedal Edema?	154
127.	Wound Bed Preparation	155
128.	Evolution of Time Frame Work	156

129.	Tissue Management Debridement	157
130.	Selection of Types of Debridement	158
131.	Types of Debridement	159
132.	Callus Debridement in Diabetic Foot	162
133.	Adhesive Felt for Offloading	164
134.	Pressure Relief Gel Pads and Support	165
135.	Deformed but Walkable Diabetic Feet	166
136.	Vacuum-assisted Wound Closure	167
137.	Footwear in Diabetes	170
138.	Footwear Insole	171
139.	Total Contact Orthosis	173
140.	Rocker Outsole	174
141.	Pathology Causing Toe Injuries due to Deformities and Poor Foot Care/Footwear	175
142.	Guidelines for Footwear Prescription in Diabetes	176
143.	Why Early Detection and Treatment of Critical Limb Ischemia	180
144.	Fungal Infection in Diabetic Foot	181
145.	Ten Commandments of Foot Care in Diabetes	182

Wound Care Mini: Glossary	183
Further Reading	187

Section 1

Medical Aspect of Diabetic Foot

Diabetes Mellitus—A Clinical Challenge

- Diabetes is a serious chronic disease that needs urgent attention
- It affects rich and poor, young and old, and developed and developing countries in equal measure
- In 2017, the global prevalence of diabetes was estimated at 424.9 million
- This figure is predicted globally to reach 628.6 million by 2045
- The majority (80%) of persons with diabetes live in low and middle-income countries
- Africa – total number of diabetes 16 million in 2017 will increase to 40.7 million by 2045
- South East Asia – total number of diabetes 82 million will increase to 151.4 million by 2045
- Middle East and North Africa – total number of diabetes 38.7 million will increase to 82 million by 2045
- Europe – total number of diabetics 58 million will increase to 66.7 million by 2045
- Western Pacific – total number of diabetics 158.8 million will increase to 185.3 million by 2045
- North America and Caribbean – total number of diabetes 45.9 million will increase to 62.7 million by 2045
- South and Central America – total number of diabetes 26 million will increase to 42.3 million by 2045.

Top Ten Countries for Number of Adults with Diabetes

No.	Countries in 2017	Total number in million	Countries in 2045	Total number in million
1	China	114.4	India	134.3
2	India	72.9	China	119.8
3	United States	30.2	United States	35.6
4	Brazil	12.5	Mexico	21.8
5	Mexico	12.0	Brazil	20.3
6	Indonesia	10.3	Egypt	16.7
7	Russian Federation	8.5	Indonesia	16.7
8	Egypt	8.2	Pakistan	16.1
9	Germany	7.5	Bangladesh	13.7
10	Pakistan	7.5	Turkey	11.2

Epidemiology of the Diabetic Foot

- Every 20 second a limb is lost due to diabetes
- Approximately 15% of all people with diabetes will be affected by a foot ulcer during their lifetime
- Five year recurrence rates of ulcer are 70%
- Up to 85% of amputations in relation to people with diabetes are preceded by a foot ulcer
- People with diabetes with one lower limb amputation have a 50% risk of developing a serious lesion in the second limb within 2 years
- People with diabetes have a 50% mortality rate in the 5 years following the initial amputation
- Across the globe, 40–60% of all lower extremity nontraumatic amputations
- Foot complications, especially serious ones like the septic limb, can be serious and costly
- 85% of all diabetic foot related problems are preventable.

Economical Burden of the Diabetic Foot Ulcer

- Diabetic foot complications are expensive due to:
  - Frequent visits to clinic
  - Prolonged and frequent hospitalization
  - Investigations—laboratory tests, etc.
  - Medications
  - Surgeries
  - Off loading devices
  - Specialized foot wear
  - Rehabilitation
  - Increased need for home-care
  - Absent from work
- Given the high cost of diabetic foot ulcers and amputations to both the individual and society, the relatively low cost interventions of foot-care are likely to be cost-effective in most societies.

Pathway to Diabetic Foot Ulcer

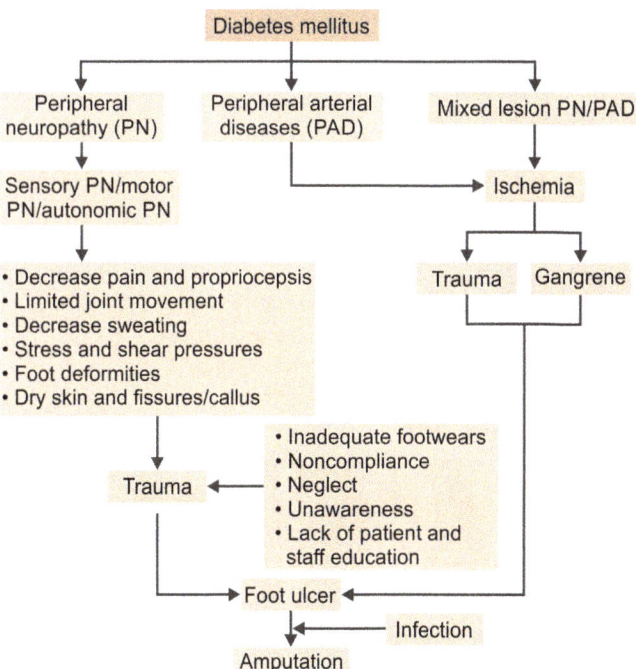

Factors Associated with Foot Ulcer

Peripheral neuropathy	Sensorimotor/autonomic
Peripheral arterial disease	
Trauma	Poor footwear • Walking barefoot • Falls/accidents • Objects inside shoes
Biomechanics	Limited joint mobility • Bony prominence • Foot deformity/osteoarthropathy • Callus
Socioeconomic status	Low socioeconomic position • Poor access to health care • Noncompliance neglect • Poor education
Previous ulcer/amputation	

Callus	Deformity	Blister	Bare foot –burn

Bullae	Charcot	Herbal	Rat Bite

Pathophysiology of Foot Ulceration

Complex interplay of various factors includes:
- Peripheral neuropathy (the most important cause of diabetic foot ulcer):
  - Sensory
  - Motor
  - Autonomic
- Peripheral arterial diseases
- Neuroischemic ulcers (mixed group)
- Infection
- Nonulcerative lesions
- Trauma
- Biomechanics factors
- Cultural and socioeconomic factors
- Health care workers (training, skills, etc.).

Diabetic Peripheral Neuropathy

- Sensorimotor and autonomic are major risk factors for diabetic foot ulcers
- Neuropathy cannot be diagnosed by history alone; a careful foot examination is mandatory
- Up to 50% of type 2 diabetic patients have significant neuropathy and "at-risk" feet
- Associated with loss of sensation - sequel include the following:
  - Callosities, crack soles
  - Break down of skin, burn, nondiscernible injury (e.g., rat bites)
  - All these may lead to infection, morbidity, and mortality.

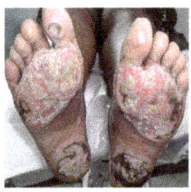
Sensory neuropathy

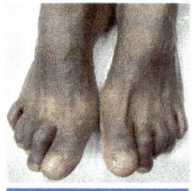
Motor neuropathy

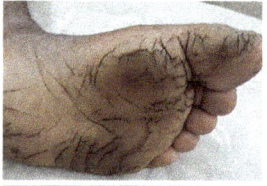
Autonomic neuropathy

Types of Peripheral Neuropathy

Etiology	Sensory neuropathy 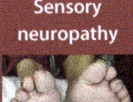	Autonomic neuropathy 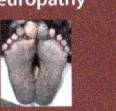	Motor neuropathy 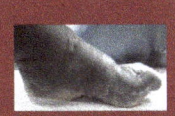
Characteristics	<ul><li>Loss of protective sensation</li><li>No perception of shoes rubbing or temperature changes</li></ul>	<ul><li>Reduce sweating results in dry cracked skin</li><li>Increased blood flow leads to a warm foot</li></ul>	<ul><li>Dysfunction of the motor nerves that control the movement of the foot</li><li>Limited joint mobility may increase plantar pressure</li><li>Foot deformities develop</li><li>Hammer toes</li></ul>
Clinical presentations	<ul><li>Unaware of a foot ulcer or lack of discomfort when a wound is being probed</li></ul>	<ul><li>Dry skin with cracks and fissures</li><li>Bounding pulses</li><li>Dilated dorsal veins</li><li>Warm feet</li></ul>	<ul><li>High medial longitudinal arch, leading to prominent metatarsal heads and pressure points over the plantar forefoot.</li><li>Clawed toes</li><li>Altered gait</li></ul>

Tests for Peripheral Neuropathy

Semmes Weinstein Monofilament

- The 10 g monofilament (5.07) testing is recommended as a screening tool to determine the presence of protective sensation in persons with diabetes.

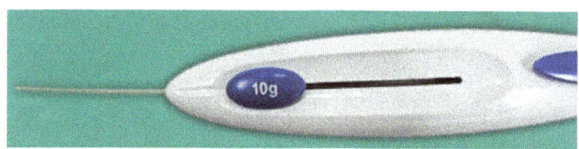

Places for Testing

- *Big toe, #3rd toe and 5th toe
- Plantar surface of the metatarsal heads (*1st, 3rd, and #5th metatarsal heads)
- The medial and lateral sides of the plantar aspect of the mid foot
- The plantar area of the heel
- The dorsal aspect of the mid foot.

*Recommended by International Working Group of Diabetic Foot
#Others are options.

Vibration Test

128 Hz Turning Fork

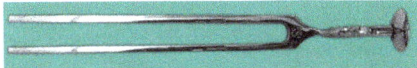

Vibra-Tip

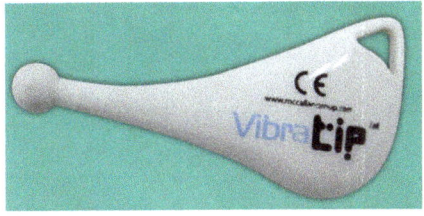

A pocket-sized, wipe-clean, battery operated disposable device for checking vibration sensation.

Biothesiometer or Neuro-esthesiometer

These instruments (e.g., biothesiometer or neuro-esthesiometer) are too expensive for many centers.

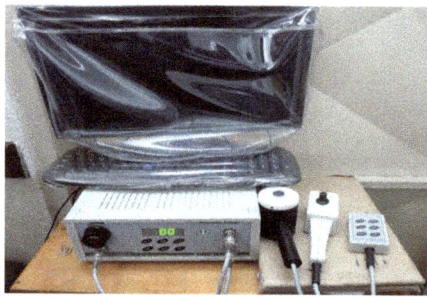

Other Tests for Peripheral Neuropathy

Tender Hammer
- Tender reflex for deep sensation.

Temperature Test
- Tip thermal for temperature test.

Cotton Test
- Touch of a cotton wool for touch test.

Pain Test
- Pain test with toothpick.

Neuropad (Autonomic Test)

- A simple visual indicator test to evaluate sympathetic autonomic neuropathy (sweating) in the feet
- Predicts risk of foot ulceration.

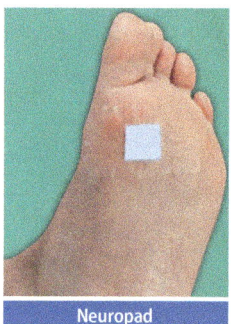

Neuropad

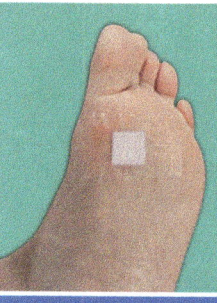

No autonomic neuropathy – sweating and color change of the Neuropad

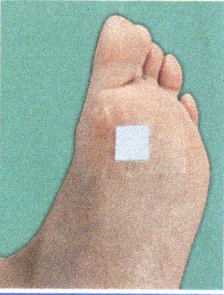

Autonomic neuropathy – no sweating and no color change of the Neuropad

Neuro-osteoarthropathy (Charcot Foot)

- Neuropathic bone and joint disease sometimes referred to as a "Charcot-foot" (neuro-osteoarthropathic)
- Among the most devastating diabetic foot complication
- Symptoms usually include a hot, erythematous swollen foot, possible pain, usually no break in the skin, and no radiographic changes
- Rapid progression with bone fragmentation and destruction of joints
- Etiology of this process is not known
- Neuropathy and good bounding pulses are usually present
- Precipitating trauma is often reported
- Clear differentiation from infection is important to avoid misdiagnosed and possible amputation
- Treatment is empirical at present includes total contact casting and limitation of activity
- Suspected Charcot foot requires specialized attention and should always be referred to specialized center.

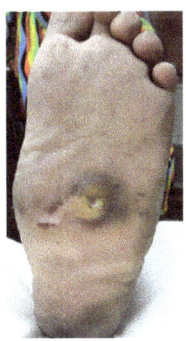

Indications for a Neurological Referral in Patients with Suspected Diabetic Sensorimotor Neuropathy

Asymmetrical signs

- Predominant motor signs
- Rapid progression of symptoms/signs
- Back or neck pain
- Family history of neuropathy
- Any suggestion of chronic inflammatory demyelinating neuropathy

Oral Symptomatic Therapies in Painful Diabetic Neuropathy

Drug class	Drug	Daily dose (mg)
Tricyclic antidepressants	Amitriptyline	10–150
	Imipramine	10–150
SNRIs	Duloxetine	60–120
Anticonvulsants	Gabapentin	900–3,600
	Pregabalin	150–600
Opioids	Tramadol	50–400
	Oxycodone CR	10–60

SNRIs—serotonin and noradrenaline reuptake inhibitors.

Peripheral Arterial Diseases

- Peripheral arterial disease is the most important factor related to outcome of a diabetic foot ulcer
- Peripheral arterial disease can often be recognized by simple clinical examination: Color and temperature of the skin, palpation of pedal pulses, and ankle blood pressure measurement
- The probability of a diabetic foot ulcer healing can be estimated using noninvasive vascular tests. Ankle and occasionally toe blood pressure readings may be falsely elevated due to medial sclerosis
- Rest pain due to ischemia may be absent in diabetic patients (probably) due to peripheral neuropathy
- Conservatives approaches should involve a walking program (if no ulcer or gangrene is present), appropriate foot wear, cessation of smoking, and aggressive treatment of hypertension and dyslipidemia
- Patency rates and limb salvage rates after revascularization do not differ between diabetic and nondiabetic patient; therefore, diabetic is not a reason to withhold this treatment.

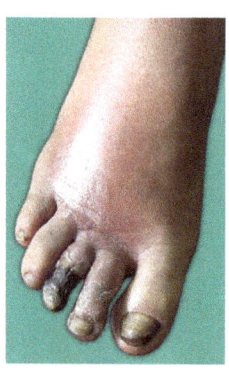

Stages of Peripheral Arterial Disease

The Fontaine classification is a method by which peripheral artery disease is clinically classified. Peripheral artery disease may be asymptomatic or symptomatic and the spectrum of symptoms is classified according to the Fontaine classification.

Stage I: Asymptomatic occlusive arterial disease without clinical symptoms.
Stage II: Intermittent claudication. This stage takes into account the fact that patients usually have a very constant distance at which they have pain:

- Stage IIa: Intermittent claudication after more than 200 meters of pain free walking
- Stage IIb: Intermittent claudication after less than 200 meters of walking

Stage III: Rest pain. Ischemic rest pain is especially troubling for patients during the night.

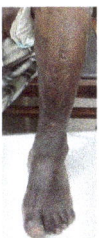

Stage IV: Ischemic ulcers or gangrene.

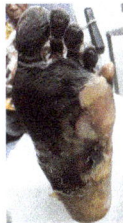 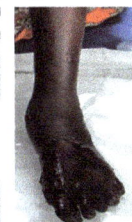 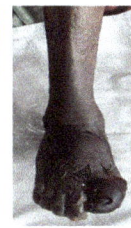

Chronic Critical Ischemia

This is chronic manifestation of peripheral arterial disease where arteries of lower limbs are severely blocked.
Chronic critical ischemia has been defined by either of the two following criteria:

- Persistent ischemic rest pain requiring regular analgesia for more than two weeks
- Ulceration or gangrene of the foot or toes
- Both associated with low ankle systolic pressure.

If left untreated it will results in amputation of the affected limb.

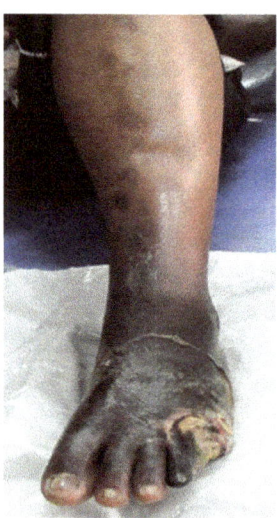 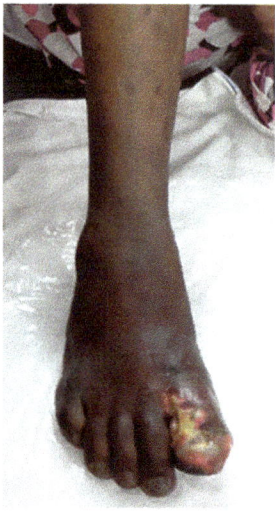

Classification of Peripheral Arterial Disease

Grade 1: No symptoms or signs of peripheral arterial disease (PAD) in the effected foot with:
- Palpable dorsalis pedal and posterior tibial artery
- Ankle-brachial index 0.9–1.0
- Toe brachial Index ABI >0.6 or transcutaneous oxygen pressure ($TcPO_2$) >60 mm Hg.

Grade 2: Symptoms or signs of PAD, but not of critical limb ischemia
- Presence of intermittent claudication
- Ankle-brachial index <0.9, but ankle pressure >50 mm Hg
- Toe brachial index <0.6, systolic toe blood pressure >30 mm Hg
- $TcPO_2$ 30–60 mm Hg
- Other abnormalities on noninvasive testing compatible with PAD.

Grade 3: Critical limb ischemia
- Systolic ankle blood pressure <50 mm Hg
- Systolic toe blood pressure <30 mm Hg
- $TcPO_2$ <30 mm Hg.

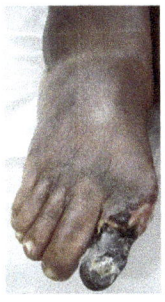

Interpretation of the Ankle-brachial Index

Ankle-brachial index	Interpretation
>1.30	Poorly compressible vessels, arterial calcification
0.90–1.30	Normal
0.60–0.89	Mild arterial obstruction
0.40–0.59	Moderate obstruction
<0.40	Severe obstruction

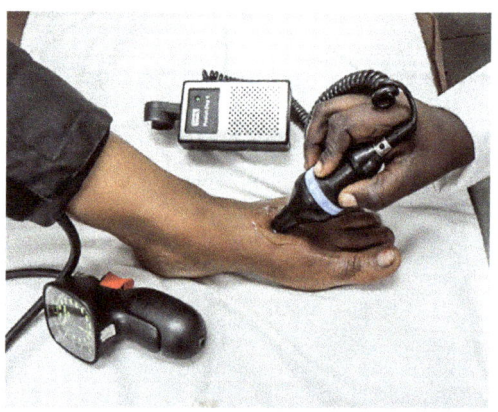

Computed Tomography Scan Angiogram of Lower Limbs

- Computed tomography angiography are quite comparable in visualizing vessels
- Computed tomography angiogram in patients with poor vascularity
- It is done to evaluate the extend of arterial block
- Helps the feasibility of revascularization.

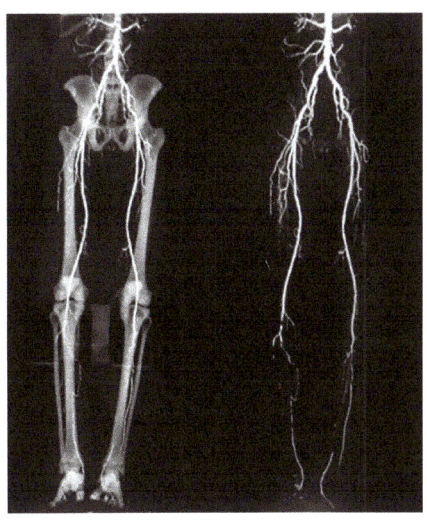

Transcutaneous Oxygen Monitor

Transcutaneous oxygen ($TcPO_2$/TCOM) measures the local oxygen released from the skin through the capillaries, reflecting the metabolic state of the lower limb.

Transcutaneous oxygen is noninvasive monitoring of oxygen tension on the skin.

Used in several clinical situation:

- Diagnosis of ischemia
- Wound management
- Qualification for hyperbaric oxygen therapy
- Revascularization
- Predicting limb amputation
- Level of amputation.

Clinical Symptoms of Neuropathic and Ischemic Foot Ulcers

Clinical signs	Neuropathic ulcer	Ischemic ulcer
Skin color	Normal or red	Pale/bluish. Pronounced redness when lowered (dependent rubor), blanching on elevation
Skin condition	Dry skin, fissure, and cracks due to decreased sweating	Thin, fragile, and dry skin
Callus present	Commonly seen on the weight-bearing areas and is generally thick	Not usually, if present, distal eschar or necrosis
Foot deformities	Clawed toes, possible high arch, possible Charcot deformities.	No specific deformities. Possible absent toes/forefoot from previous amputations
Ulcer location	On the plantar aspects of the foot/toes/heel	Distal/tips of the toes, heel, lateral boarder of the foot
Ulcer characteristics	Usually painless, with a "punched out" appearance (granulation or deeper base) surrounded by callus	Painful, especially with necrosis or slough with poor granulation

Contd...

Contd...

Clinical signs	Neuropathic ulcer	Ischemic ulcer
Sensation	Reduced or absent sensation to touch, vibration, pain, and pressure	Painful sensation may be present but decreased if there is associated neuropathy
Ankle reflexes	Usually not present	Usually present
Foot temperature	Warm	Cold or decreased temperature
Foot pulses	Present and often bounding. Dilated, prominent veins	Absent or markedly reduced

Neuroischemic Diabetic Foot (Mixed)

The Neuroischemic Diabetic Foot

These two situations, which are also defined as neuropathic foot or ischemic foot, are deeply different from each other. however, in most patients who are mainly of age, both neuropathy and vasculopathy coexist: This is when we talk about neuroischemic foot.

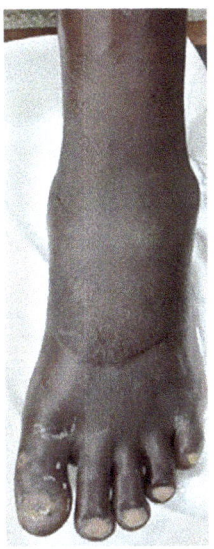

Diabetic Foot Infections

- Infection in a diabetic foot is limb-threatening and must be treated empirically and aggressively
- Signs and symptoms of infection [fever, increased white blood count, elevated erythrocyte sedimentation rate (ESR)] may often be absent in diabetic patients with infected foot ulcers
- A superficial infection is usually caused by Gram-positive bacteria, whereas deep infections are often polymicrobial, involving anaerobic and Gram-negative bacteria
- In acute deep foot infection, surgical removal of infected tissue is essential
- A multidisciplinary approach providing debridement, meticulous wound care, adequate vascular supply, metabolic control, empirical antimicrobial treatment, and relief of pressure is essential in the treatment of foot infection.

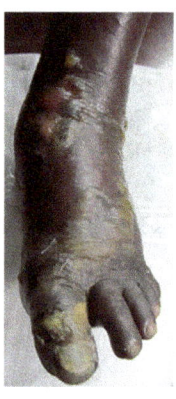

Risk Factors for Infection

Factors increase the risk of infection one should be aware of that increase likelihood of infection:
- A history of bare foot walking
- Loss of protective sensation
- The presence of renal insufficiency
- A traumatic foot wound
- Presence of peripheral arterial disease in the affected limb
- Diabetic foot ulcer present for more than 30 days
- History of recurrent diabetic foot ulcers
- A positive probe to bone test
- A previous lower extremity amputation.

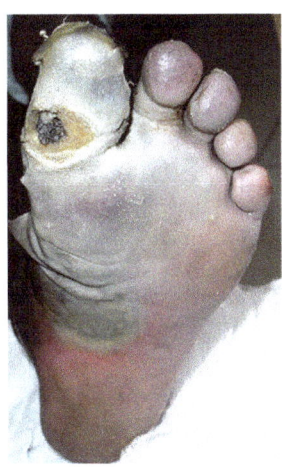

Three Most Important Clinical Categories of Infections

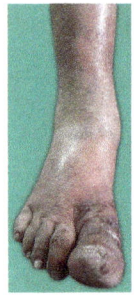

- Cellulitis (the least invasive infection)

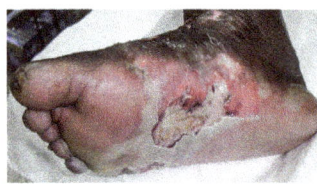

- Deep soft tissue infection (involve fascia, muscles, tendons)

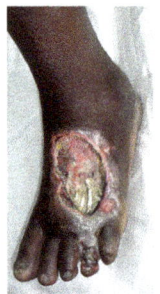

- Chronic osteomyelitis (involves bone).

Cellulitis

- Most common foot problem
- Characterized by erythema, swelling, heat, and lymphangitis may be present
- No ulcer or wound exudates is present
- Surgical debridement not required.

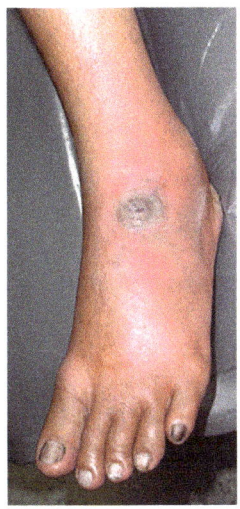

Deep Soft Tissue Infection

- Patient may be acutely sick
- Involves deeper structure
- Crepitation may be noted over the afflicted area
- Discharge if present is often foul smelling
- Necrotizing may be life threatening
- Debridement can be life saving.

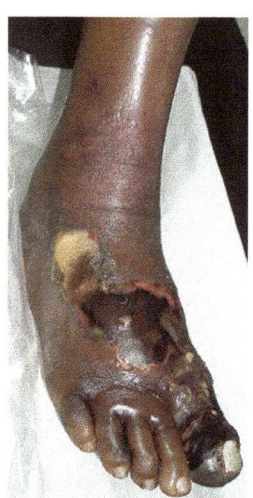

Chronic Osteomyelitis

- The specter of osteomyelitis haunts the management of the diabetic foot
- Both lay persons and health care professionals have a strong sense that when infection is in the bone the prospects for successful treatment are low
- Osteomyelitis is one of the end stages on the path to amputation reputation for intractability and recurrence
- Temperature is usually less
- Discharge is commonly foul
- No lymphangitis is observed
- Pain may or may not be depending degree of peripheral neuropathy
- Deep penetrating ulcers and sinus tract.

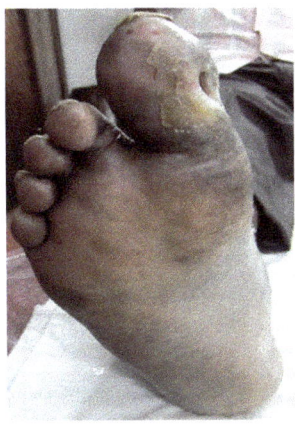
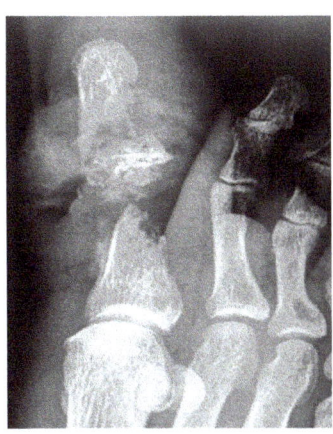

Criteria for Diagnosis of Osteomyelitis

The following criteria can be used for the diagnosis of osteomyelitis, which is likely when three criteria are positive and an ulcer is present.
- Cellulitis
- Probing to bone
- Positive bacteriological culture from deep tissue
- Radiological and/or computed tomography scan compatible with osteitis
- Histological diagnosis.

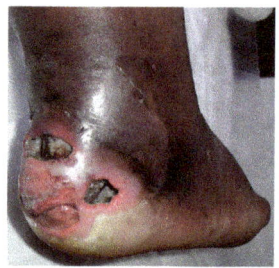

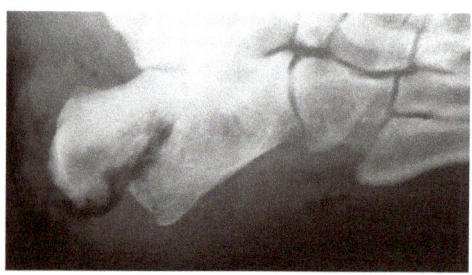

Typical Features of Diabetic Foot Osteomyelitis on Plain X-rays

- Periosteal reaction or elevation
- Loss of bone cortex with bony erosion
- Focal loss of cortical trabecular pattern or marrow radiolucency
- Bone sclerosis, with or without erosion
- Presence of sequestrum: Devitalized bone with radio-dense appearance that has become separated from normal bone
- Presence of involucrum: A layer of new bone growth outside previously existing bone resulting from stripping off of the periosteum and new bone growing from the periosteum.

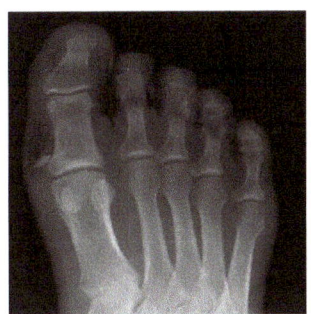 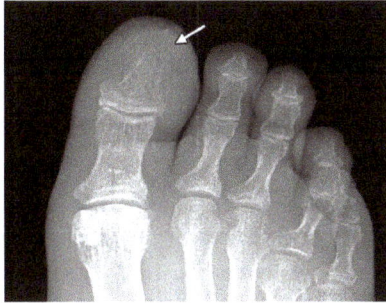

Classification and Severity of Infection

Once it is confirmed diagnosis of a diabetic foot infection, define both the presence and severity of infection.

The classification systems for defining the presence and severity of an infection:

Clinical criteria	Grade/severity
No clinical signs of infection	Grade 1/uninfected
Superficial tissue lesion with at least two of the following signs: • Local warmth • Erythema >0.5–2 cm around the ulcer • Local tenderness/pain • Local swelling/induration • Purulent discharge Other causes of inflammation of the skin must be excluded	Grade 2/mild
Erythema >2 cm and one of the findings above or: • Infection involving structures beneath the skin/subcutaneous tissue (e.g., deep abscess, lymphangitis, osteomyelitis, septic arthritis, fasciitis) • No systemic inflammation response as below	Grade 3/moderate
Presence of systemic signs with atleast two of the followings: • Temperature >38°C or <36°C • Pulse >90 beats per minute • Respiratory rate >20/minute • $PaCO_2$ <32 mm Hg • White cell count 12,000 mm^3 or <4,000 mm^3 • 10% immature leukocytes	Grade 4/severe

Indications of Worsening Infection

Signs and symptoms	• Drainage, erythema, temperature
	• Swelling, foul smell, fever with chills
	• Superficial bullae
	• Petechial hemorrhages, ecchymosis
	• Fluctuance and soft tissue crepitus
	• Lymphangitis and lymphadenopathy
	• Gangrene
	• Tachycardia, orthostatic hypotension
	• Delirium, stupor
Laboratory tests	• ↑ Total leukocyte count, ESR ↑
	• CRP ↑
	• Plasma glucose and HbA1c ↑
	• Ketones in serum and urine electrolyte abnormalities, worsening azotemia
Radiological investigations (X-ray foot)	• Gas in the soft tissue
	• Osteomyelitis

ESR, erythrocyte sedimentation rate; CRP, C-reactive protein; HbA1c, glycosylated hemoglobin.

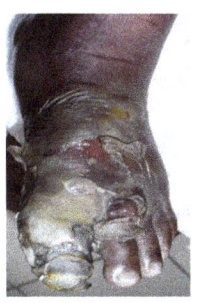

Characteristics Suggesting a More Serious Diabetic Foot Infection and Potential Indications for Hospitalization

Findings Suggesting a More Serious Diabetic Foot Infection

Wound specific	
Wound	Penetrate to subcutaneous tissue (e.g., fascia, tendon, muscle, joint, bone)
Cellulitis	Extensive (>2 cm), distance from ulceration or rapidly progressive
Local signs	Severe inflammation or induration, crepitus bullae, discoloration, necrosis or gangrene, ecchymoses or petechiae, new anesthesia
General	
Presentation	Acute onset/worsening or rapidly progressive
Systemic signs	Fever, chills, hypotension, confusion, volume depletion
Laboratory tests	Leukocytosis, very high C-reactive protein or erythrocyte sedimentation rate, severe/worsening azotemia, electrolyte abnormalities
Complicating features	Presence of a foreign body (accidental or surgically implanted), punctured wound, deep abscess, arterial or venous insufficiency, lymphedema, immunosuppressive illness or treatment
Current treatment	Progression while on apparently appropriate antibiotics supportive therapy

Factors Suggested Hospitalization may be Necessary

- Severe infection
- Metabolic or hemodynamic instability
- Intravenous therapy needed (not available/appropriate as outpatient)
- Diagnostic tests needed that are not available as outpatient
- Critical foot ischemia present
- Surgical procedures (more than minor) required
- Failure of outpatient management
- Patient unable or unwilling to comply with outpatient-based treatment
- Need for more complex dressing changes than patients/caregivers can provide
- Need for careful continuous observation.

Factors that May Influence Choices of Antibiotics Therapy for Diabetic Foot Infections (Specific Agents, Route of Administration, Duration of Therapy)

Infection Related
- Clinical severity of the infection
- History of antibiotics therapy within three months
- Presence of bone infection.

Pathogen Related
- Depends on the report of culture and sensitivity
- Depends on the outcome of bed-side Gram-staining.

Patient Related
- Pregnant/lactating women
- Allergy to any antibiotics
- Impaired immunological status patient adherence to therapy
- Impaired gastrointestinal absorption
- Peripheral arterial disease in affected limb
- High risk of unusual pathogens.

Drug Related
- Safety profile
- Drug interaction
- Frequency of dosing
- Formula availability/restriction
- Cost consideration
- Approval for indication
- Likelihood of inducing
- Publish efficacy data.

Factors Potentially Favoring Selecting Either Primarily Antibiotics or Surgical Resection for Diabetic Foot Osteomyelitis

Medical

- Patient is too medically unstable for surgery
- Poor postoperatively mechanics of foot is likely
- No other surgical procedures on foot are needed
- Infection is confined to small, forefoot lesion
- No adequate skilled surgeon is available
- Surgery cost are prohibitive for the patients
- Patient has a strong preference to avoid surgery.

Surgical

- Foot infection is associated with substantial bone necrosis or exposed joint
- Foot appears to be functionally nonsalvageable
- Patient is already nonambulatory
- Patient is at particular high risk for antibiotics related problems
- Infecting pathogens is resistant to available antibiotics
- Limb has uncorrectable ischemia (precluding systemic antibiotics delivery)
- Patient has a strong preference for surgical treatment.

Antibiotic Regimens for Mild, Moderate, and Severe Diabetic Foot Infections

Table 1

Mild diabetic foot infection		
Cephalexin	500 mg orally	QID
Amoxicillin/clavulanate	875/125 mg orally	BID
Moxifloxacin	400 mg orally	OD
Levofloxacin	500 mg orally	OD
Methicillin-resistant *Staphylococcus aureus*		
Doxycycline	100 mg orally	BID
Trimethoprim/sulfamethoxazole	160/800 mg orally	BID

IV, intravenous; QID, four times a day; OD, once daily; TDS, thrice a day; BID, twice a day.

Table 2

Moderate diabetic foot infection		
Ampicillin/sulbactam	3 g IV	QID
Ceftriaxone +	1–2 g IV	OD
Metronidazole	500 mg IV	TDS
Levofloxacin	500 mg IV	OD
Moxifloxacin	400 mg IV	OD
Ertapenem	1 g IV	OD
Cefotaxime	1 g IV	BID
Imipenem-cilastatin	500 mg IV	TDS
Methicillin-resistant *Staphylococcus aureus*		
Linezolid	600 mg in 300 mL	BID
Daptomycin	4 mg/kg IV	OD
Cefazolin	1–2 g IV	TDS

IV, intravenous; QID, four times a day; TDS, thrice a day; BID, twice a day; OD, once daily.

Table 3

Severe diabetic foot infection		
Ciprofloxacin +	400 mg IV	BID
Piperacillin/tazobactam	4 g + 0.5 g IV	TDS
Imipenem/cilastatin	500 mg IV	TDS
Tigecycline	100 mg IV loading dose then 50 mg IV	BID
Vancomycin +	30 mg/kg IV	BID
Ciprofloxacin +	400 mg IV	BID
Metronidazole	500 mg IV	TDS
Methicillin-resistant *Staphylococcus aureus*		
Linezolid	600 mg IV	BID
Daptomycin	4 mg/kg IV	OD
Tigecycline	100 mg IV loading dose then 50 mg IV	BID
Pseudomonas aeruginosa		
Piperacillin-tazobactam	4 g + 0.5 g IV	TDS

IV, intravenous; OD, once daily; BID, twice a day; TDS, thrice a day.

Duration of Treatment for Infected Diabetic Foot

Type of infection	Treatment	Duration of treatment
Uninfected ulcers	Do not require antibiotics therapy	
Mild infections	Semisynthetic penicillin (amoxicillin clavulanate, cloxacillin, flucloxacillin) or cephalosporins. Treat on as an outpatient basis unless contradiction or need arise	1–2 weeks is usually enough
Moderate infections	Broad spectrum coverage if urgently empiric antibiotics therapy required. Appropriate choices include carbapenem-class antimicrobials (ertapenem, imipenem or a penicillin/penicillinase inhibitor (e.g., piperacillin-tazobactam, ampicillin-sulbactam, or amoxicillin clavulanate), and combination of anaerobes like metronidazole or orinadazole and combinations of cephalosporins If previous history or high degree of suspicion for infection with methicillin-resistant *Staphylococcus aureus*, then consider oxazolidinone-class (linezolid)	2–6 weeks (if no bone involvement)

Contd...

Contd...

Type of infection	Treatment	Duration of treatment
	Hospitalization may be required for surgical intervention	
Severe infections	Similar to above, but must be treated urgently with initial hospitalization and intravenous antibiotics	2–8 weeks depends on the nature of any surgery and the presence of bacteremia
Osteomyelitis	Diagnosis difficult. Treatment requires consideration for both surgical resection of infected or necrotic bone and antimicrobial therapy or, in some cases, suppressive antimicrobial therapy alone	All involved bone is removed (surgically) treatment based on soft tissue involvement; if uninfected, prophylaxis for up to 72 hours; if infected treat for 4 weeks
		Infected but viable bone remains 4–6 weeks
		Dead bone remains: Minimum of 6–12 weeks (long time antibiotics regimes are sometimes used to suppress, rather than attempt to cure, infection)

Wagner Classification

Grade	Ulcer appearance
Grade 0	No open lesion; may have deformity or cellulitis
Grade 1	Superficial diabetic ulcer (partial or full thickness)
Grade 2	Ulcer extension to ligament, tendon, joint capsule, or deep fascia without abscess or osteomyelitis
Grade 3	Deep ulcer with abscess, osteomyelitis, or joint sepsis
Grade 4	Gangrene localized to portion of forefoot or heel
Grade 5	Extensive gangrenous involvement of the entire foot

PEDIS Classification

P–Perfusion

Grade 1: No symptoms or signs of peripheral arterial disease with palpable dorsal pedis and posterior tibial artery or ankle-brachial index (ABI) between 0.9-1.10 or toe brachial indices (TBI) >0.6 or transcutaneous oxygen pressure ($TcPO_2$) >60 mm Hg

Grade 2: Symptoms or signs of peripheral arterial disease (PAD) present, but not of critical limb ischemia Presence of intermittent claudication or ABI <0.9, but with ankle pressure >50 mm Hg, TBI <0.6, but systolic toe blood pressure >30 mm Hg or $TcPO_2$ 30–60 mm Hg or other abnormalities on non-invasive testing, compatible with PAD

Grade 3: Critical limb ischemia as defined by Systolic ankle blood pressure <50 mm Hg or systolic toe blood pressure <30 mm Hg or $TcPO_2$ <30 mm Hg.

E–Extent/Wound size

Wound size after debridement.

D–Depth/Tissue size

Grade 1: Superficial full thickness ulcer, not penetrating any structure deeper than the dermis

Grade 2: Deep ulcer penetrating below the dermis to subcutaneous structures involving fascia, muscles, or tendon

Grade 3: All subsequently layers of the foot involved, including bone and or joint.

I–Infection

Grade 1: No infection

Grade 2: Infection involving the skin and subcutaneous tissue only. At least two of the following items are present: local swelling or induration: Erythema >0.05 to 2 cm around the ulcer, local tenderness or pain, local warmth, purulent discharge. No systemic signs, as describe below

Grade 3: Erythema >2 cm plus one of the items describe above, or infection involving structure deeper than skin and subcutaneous tissue such as abscess, osteomyelitis, septic arthritis, fasciitis. No systemic signs

Grade 4: Any foot infection with two or more of the following condition: Temperature >38°C or <36°C, heart rate >90 beats/min >12,000 or <4,000/mm^3, >10% immature (band) forms.

S–Sensations

Grade 1: No loss of protective sensation on the affected foot

Grade 2: Loss of protective sensation on the affected foot, defined as the absence of perception in the affected foot to pressure (10 g monofilament) or vibration.

The University of Texas Classification

Depth	Grades	0	1	2	3
		Skin intact	Superficial	Deep not involving bone or joint	Involved bone or joint
A	Neither infected nor ischemic				
B	Infected but not ischemic				
C	Ischemic but not infected				
D	Both infected and ischemic				

SINDBAD Classification

Category	Definition	SINBAD score
Site	Forefoot	0
	Midfoot and hindfoot	1
Ischemia	Pedal blood flow intact: At least one pulse palpable	0
	Clinical evidence of reduced pedal blood flow	1
Neuropathy	Protective sensation intact	0
	Protective sensation lost	1
Bacterial infection	None	0
	Present	1
Area	Ulcer <1 cm^2	0
	Ulcer ≥1 cm^2	1
Depth	Ulcer confined to skin and subcutaneous tissue	0
	Ulcer reaching muscle, tendon, or deeper	1
Total possible score		6

Lower Extremity Threatened Limb Classification System

Risk stratification is based on three major factors (wound, ischemia, and infection) that impact amputation risk and clinical management.

WIFI Classification

W = Wound : Extent and depth
I = Ischemia : Perfusion flow of blood
FI = Foot infection : Presence and extent of infection.

Wound—Clinical Category

Grade	Clinical description
0	Ischemic rest pain; Pre-gangrenous skin change, without frank ulcer or gangrene (PEDIS or UT Class 0)
1	Minor tissue loss: Small shallow ulceration) <5 cm^2 on foot or distal leg (PEDIS or UT Class 1); no exposed bone unless limited to distal phalanx
2	Major tissue loss: Deeper ulceration(s) with exposed bone, joint or tendon, ulcer 5–10 cm^2 not involving calcaneus – (PEDIS or UT Classes 2 and 3); gangrenous changes limited to digits. Salvageable with multiple digital amps or standard tower mounted amplifiers (TMAs) + skin coverage
3	Extensive ulcer/gangrene >10 cm^2 involving forefoot or mid foot; full thickness heel ulcer >5 cm^2 + calcaneal involvement. Salvageable only with complex foot reconstruction, nontraditional TMA (Chopart/Lisfranc); flap coverage or complex wound management needed

Ischemia: Clinical Category

Grade	ABI	Ankle SP	TP, TcPO$_2$
0	≥0.80	≥100 mm Hg	≥60 mm Hg
1	0.60–0.79	70–99 mm Hg	40–59 mm Hg
2	0.40–0.59	50–69 mm Hg	30–39 mm Hg
3	<0.40	<50 mm Hg	<30 mm Hg

ABI, ankle-brachial index; TcPO$_2$, transcutaneous oxygen pressure; SP, systolic pressure.

Foot Infection: Clinical Category

Grade	Clinical Description
0	Wound without pus or manifestation of infection
1	>2 manifestation of infection (redness, pus, pain, tenderness, warmth, induration) any cellulitis or erythema extends <2 cm around ulcer; infection is limited to skin or subcutaneous tissues; no local complications or systemic illness
2	Infection in patient who is systemically and metabolically stable, but has >1 of the following: cellulitis extending 2 cms, lymphangitis; spread beneath fascia; deep tissue abscess; gangrene; muscles, tendon, joint or bone involvement
3	Infection in patients with systemic or metabolic toxicity

Simple Staging of the Diabetic Foot

The natural history of the diabetic foot can be divided into six stages:

Stage 1: The normal foot
- The foot is normal and patient does not have risk factors like neuropathy, ischemia, deformity, callus, etc.

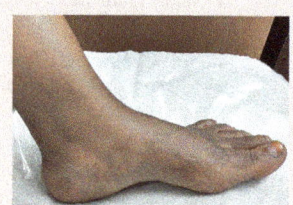

Stage 2: High risk foot
- The patient has developed one or more risk factors for the ulceration of the foot

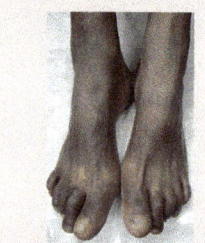

Stage 3: Foot with ulcer
- Neuropathic foot ulcers develops on plantar surface due to high mechanical pressure
- Neuro-ischemic ulcers develops on the margins of foot and toes due poorly fitting shoes

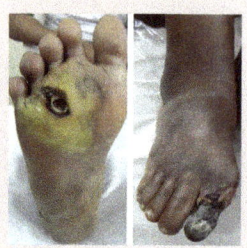

Contd...

Contd...

Stage 4: Foot with cellulitis
- The ulcer has developed infection with the presence of cellulitis can complicate both neuropathic and neuroischemic foot

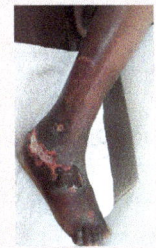

Stage 5: Foot with necrosis
- In neuropathic foot infection is the cause of necrosis
- In neuroischemic foot infection is the cause of necrosis and ischemia leads directly to necrosis

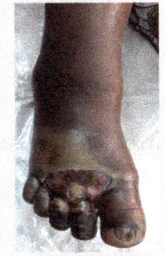

Stage 6: Unsalvageable foot presentation
- The foot cannot be saved and will need a major amputation

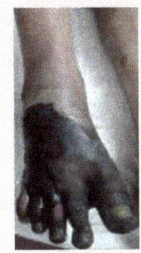

Consider the Whole Patient and not the Hole in the Patient to Ensure Effective Care of the Foot Ulcer

History of the patient and medications	Check for medication that may inhibit healing (i.e., steroids, immune suppressants)
Check for other complications	Neurological, eye, heart, kidney, vascular
Glycogenic control	Glycosylated hemoglobin <7.0% good control ≥7.0% action need to be taken
Hypertension control	≤130/80 mm Hg
Obesity control	Body mass index <25 kg/m^2
Hyperlipidemia control	Cholesterol <5.2 mmol/L (200 mg/dL)

Disclaimer: These are general guidelines. Please check local treatment recommendation applicable for your country of healthcare institution.

Foot Examination

History of the patient	• History of the patient regarding foot • Symptoms of neuropathy, peripheral arterial disease, previous ulcer(s), amputation(s)
Local skin assessment	• Swelling of the foot • Color of the skin • Temperature of the skin • Dryness and cracks of the skin • Callus formation
Neurological Examination	**Sensory:** Loss of protective sensation **Autonomic:** Lack of sweating that results in dry, cracked skin that bleeds and creates a portal of entry for bacteria **Motor:** Loss of reflexes or atrophy of muscles that leads to foot deformities
Vascular Examination	• Check for peripheral arterial disease, symptoms are often not found, but the following signs may be present: Cold feet, blanching on elevation, absent hair growth, dry shiny, and atrophic skin • Palpate and check for dorsalis pedis, posterior tibial, popliteal and femoral pulse • Measure the ankle brachial pressure index (ABI), if possible toe pressures or transcutaneous oxygen may be assessed because arterial calcification can cause falsely elevated ABI results
Deformity	• Charcot foot • Hammer toes, claw toes, bunions • Check the deformity and address inappropriately fitted shoes
Check Footwear	• Check for hard outsole • Wide toe room • Flexible upper part to accommodate for any deformity

Ulcer Assessment

Size of ulcer	Length, width, depth, and location (preferably with clinical photograph or wound tracing)
Wound bed	**Appearance** • Black (necrosis) • Yellow (slough) • Red (granulation) • Pink (epithelialization)
Signs of infection	• Evaluate the ulcer for signs of inflammation, infection, and edema • Be aware that some signs (fever, pain, and increased white blood count/erythrocyte sedimentation rate) may be absent in patients with diabetes
Exudates	• Copious • Moderate • Mild • None
Wound edge	• Advancing/nonadvancing edge • Callus and scale • Maceration • Erythema • Edema
Local pain	• Burning, pins and needles, shooting and stabbing (non-stimulus dependent)
Neuropathic pain	• Deep infection or Charcot joint

Wound Bed

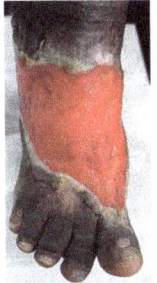
Granulation (red)

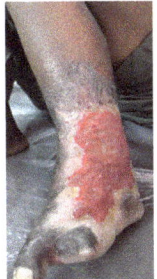
Epithelialization (pink)

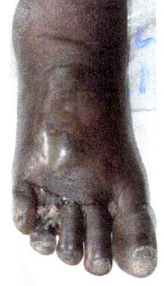
Necrosis (black)

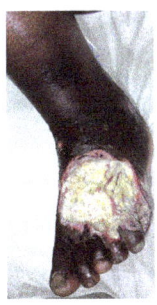
Slough (yellow)

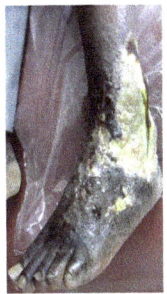
Unhealthy wound edge

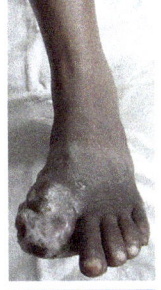
Maceration (white)

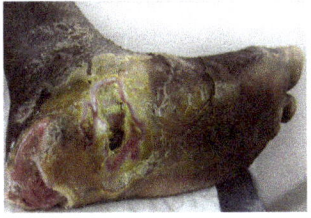
Wound undermining deep tissue infection

Examination of Edge, Wall, and Base

Healing ulcer
- Sloping edges
- Granulating clean base
- Epithelialization at edges

Chronic/static ulcer
- Straight walls/edges
- Callus at periphery
- "Pizza-like" base

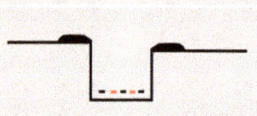

Deteriorating ulcer
- Undermined edges
- Overlying callus–often macerated
- Sloughy base ~ sinus, bone synovial fluid

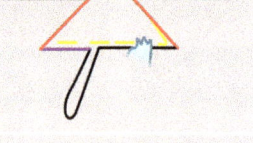

Rolled edge
- Puckered raised edge
- Evidence of nonhealing base

A Summary of the Management of Diabetic Foot Ulcer

Goal	Strategy
Improve metabolic control	• Good control of glucose helps healing
Investigations	• Regular checking of blood glucose, glycosylated hemoglobin • Full blood picture and erythrocyte sedimentation rate • Deep tissue biopsy and culture • X-ray, computed tomography scan angiography, bone scan, magnetic resonance imaging
Treat infection	Antibiotics: Oral, parenteral
Topical treatment	• Sharp debridement • Dressings • Topical agents • Skin grafting
Treat edema	• Decrease in swelling helps healing
For neuropathic pain	• Analgesic agents • Relieve anxiety
Foot surgery	• Incision/drainage • Corrective surgery • Amputation
Improve circulation	• Noninvasive vascular testing (bed side Doppler) • Percutaneous transluminal angioplasty • Vascular surgery
Offloading (decrease weight bearing)	• Removable cast walkers • Contact casting/scotch cast boot • Insoles/ortheses/forefoot orthotics • Crutches/wheelchair/bed-rest • Therapeutic footwear

Contd...

Contd...

Goal	Strategy
General condition	- Cardiovascular treatment - Hypertension, hypercholesterolemia, etc. - Treat retinopathy/nephropathy - Treat malnutrition - Cessation of smoking
Setting	- Patient/staff education - Compliance - Support/follow-up - Multidisciplinary
Organization of foot care	Minimum foot clinic combine with diabetes clinic

Local Wound Treatment

Tissue debridement	- Sharp debridement - Hydrogels alginates - Bio-surgery
Infection	Dependent on the outcomes of the wound assessment: - Topical antimicrobials (e.g., sustained silver releasing dressings) - Systemic antibiotic therapy
Exudates management	- Foams, alginates
Edge effect	- The treatment of the edge depends on the outcomes of the assessment of the edge of the wound. In general, healthy wounds have a pink wound bed and an advancing wound margin while unhealthy wounds have a dark and undermined wound margin
Neuropathic pain	Occasionally, neuropathy can be associated with pain. If pain is present, consider the following treatment, which are used: - Gabapentin, pregabalin, amitriptyline, duloxetine, nortriptyline, or desipramine, etc.

Disclaimer: These are general guidelines. Please check local treatment recommendations applicable for your country or healthcare institution.

Role of Debridement in Ulcer Management

- The role of debridement in ulcer management is one of the cornerstones therapy
- It should be seen as an integral part of wound care
- It is perhaps best seen as the most effective way of wound cleansing
- It is often referred to as wound bed preparation
- Debridement is the removal of all foreign material, devitalized tissue, slough, necrotic tissue, and occasionally healthy surrounding tissue
- The removal of healthy tissue is advocated when ulcer is undermined and the ulcer base is extensively hidden or where an abscess requires drainage
- Various debridement methods are discussed in table.

Debridement Methods and Its Characteristics

Characteristic	Dressings	Enzymes	Larvae	Surgical/sharp	Mechanical
Speed of action	🟡	🟡	🟡	🟢	🔴
Healthy tissue discrimination	🟢	🟡	🟢	🔴	🟡
Infection risk	🔴	🟢	🟢	🟢	🟡
Exudate prosuction	🔴	🔴	🔴	🟢	🟢
Skill	🟢	🟢	🟢	🟢	🟡
Treatment cost	🟡	🟡	🔴	🟢	🟡

🟢 Most appropriate   🟡 Moderate   🔴 Least appropriate

Summary of Indications for Different Dressings/Devices

Appearance of the wound	Therapeutic alternatives
Presence of black, dry necrotic tissue	• Hydrogel • Debridement
Presences of fibrin or moist necrotic tissue	• Hydrocolloid • Hydrogel, if lightly exuding • Alginate, if heavily exuding
Cavity wound or exposed bone	• Hydrocolloid gel • Hydrocellular or form pad • Negative pressure wound therapy
Heavily exuding wound	• Alginate • New generation–hydrocolloid • Hydrocellular or foam pad
Granulating wound	• Hydrocolloid • Hydrocellular or foam pad • Bioengineered tissue • Hydrofiber • Alginate
Superficial wound or dermabrasion, superficial burn, donor graft site	• Hydrocolloid • Hydrocellular or foam pad • Hydrogel • Film • Tulle and interface
Foul-smelling wound	• Charcot dressing

Ulcer Healing

Casting
- Casting/(non) removable offloading devices.

Footwear
- Shoes as a primary treatment modality to heal plantar foot wear.

Surgical offloading
- Achilles tendon lengthening
- Single or pan-metatarsal head resection
- Joint arthroplasty
- Osteotomy
- Digital flexor tendon
- Other procedures like flexor hallucis longus tendon transfer, plantar fascia release, or Achilles tenotomy.

Other Offloading Intervention
- Felted foam
- Ankle-foot orthoses.

Surgical Intervention in Severe Cases where Abnormal Pressure Distribution is Causing Persistent and Nonresolvable Ulceration

Assess for biomechanical abnormality	Outcome	Intervention and treatment
Inspect for callus and corns	Callus and corns detected	• Debride callus and corns, and review regularly to repeat this treatment • Assess footwear for suitability • Recommend regular self-monitoring for signs of change • Recommend regular application of emollient, specifically urea-based where callus is heavy
Inspect integrity of the plantar fat pad	Evidence of fat pad atrophy	• Select cushioning replacement therapy such as silicone-heel and forefoot padding
Joint range of motion: • Ankle • First metatarsophalangeal joint	• <10° dorsiflexion ankle joint • <60° dorsiflexion metatarsophalangeal joint	• Stretching program for Achilles tendon, prophylactic tendon-lengthening surgery for recalcitrant cases • Functional immobilization with orthotics or rocker sole, joint manipulation, surgery

Biomechanics Factors and Footwear

Biomechanics and Footwear

- Biomechanical abnormalities are frequently a consequence of diabetic neuropathy and lead to abnormal plantar foot pressure
- A combination of foot deformity and neuropathy increases the risk of ulcer
- Pressure relief is essential for the prevention and healing of an ulcer, as abnormal foot pressures lead to plantar ulceration
- Shoes and inserts should be inspected frequently and replaced when necessary
- A patient should never return to footwear which has caused ulceration
- Appropriated footwear (adapted to high pressure, deformities, and/or lesions present in the foot) has been associated with significantly fewer recurrences and development of ulceration.

Plantar Pressure Reduction

Casting
- Specially designed cast to take weight off from the diabetic foot ulcer.

Removable Walkers
- Removable cast walkers are boots for off-loading strategies to facilitate ulcer healing.

Footwear
- Diabetic footwear are specially designed shoes, or shoe inserts, intended to reduce the risk of foot ulcer or to offload an existing foot ulcer.

Surgical Offloading
- Metatarsal head resection effectively reduce pressure in the forefoot.

Other Offloading Devices

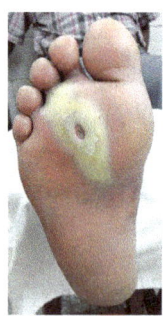
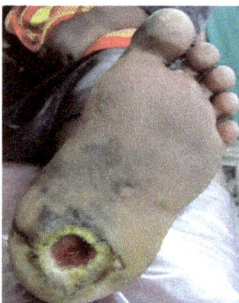
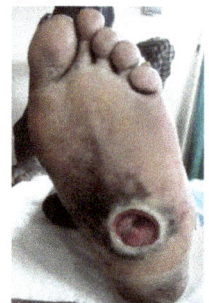

Footwear and Offloading for the Diabetic Foot: An Evidence-based Guideline

Use of footwear and off-loading techniques for the prevention and healing of plantar ulcers.
The guideline was organized around the following main outcomes:
- Ulcer prevention
- Ulcer healing
- Reduction of plantar pressure.

Selected interventions were categorized into three sub-categories:
1. Casting techniques
    - Total contact cast
    - Cast shoes
2. Footwear related techniques
    - Shoe
    - Insole
    - Orthoses (in-shoe)
    - Socks/padding
3. Other techniques
    - Bed rest
    - Crutches/wheelchair
    - Walkers
    - Off loading dressings
    - Felted foam/padding.

General Guide to Footwear Based on Risk Status

Degree of deformity	Activities		
	Low	Moderate	High
None	Sports shoe as in, or depth shoe with a soft insole	Sports or depth shoe with a thick insole	Sports or depth shoe with a thick insole; consider rocker bottom
Moderate	Sports or depth shoe with a thick insole	Sports or depth shoe with a thick insole; consider rocker bottom	Sports or depth shoe with a thick insole, rocker bottom consider custom shoe with thicker insole, consider reliefs
Severe	Customized upper or custom shoe, thick insole	Customized upper or custom shoe, thick insole with reliefs, rocker bottom	Customized upper or custom shoe, thick insole with complex reliefs, rocker bottom

Examination of the Insensate Diabetic Foot

Examination	Justification
General	Inspect for possible ulceration, areas of inflammation, other skin changes related to vascular disease
Sensory	Test vibratory sensation and perform a quantifiable sensory test to determine the level of protective sensation
Temperature	With no sensation, a localized skin temperature increase >2°C in a localized area indicates an area of inflammation
Footwear	Identify the characteristics of the footwear that may pose a threat to the feet, because of wear or style
Muscle	Diseases that result in sensory loss can also lead to muscle paralysis; in the feet, intrinsic paralysis is the most frequent early involvement and results in clawed toe deformities

The Diabetic Foot Ulcers: Outcome and Management

- In diabetes, healing of foot ulcers is limited by multiple factors and therefore requires a multifactorial approach
- Control of infection, treatment of arterial disease, pressure relief, and wound management are essential components of the multifactorial treatment of foot ulcers
- Type, site, and cause of the ulcer must be considered in choosing treatment strategies
- Topical wound management is adjunctive to systematic and surgical treatment
- Continuity of care and lifelong observation of the diabetic foot at risk are essential both in management and prevention of foot ulcers.

Global Burden of Limb Amputation

- Every 20 seconds a limb is lost due to diabetes
- One million limb amputation occur yearly in people with diabetes
- Patients with diabetes are 40 times likely to lose a limb than nondiabetes
- 70% of all limbs amp happens to people with diabetes
- Five years mortality after limb amputation is 70% in people with diabetes
- Contralateral limb amputation rate in 50% in 5 years in people with diabetes
- Life time risk of foot ulcer in patients with diabetes is 15%
- 85% of the limbs amputation is preceded by minor foot lesions.

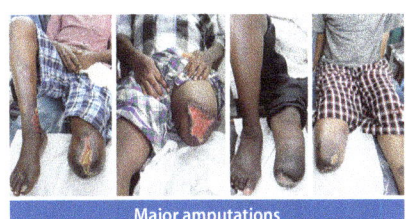

Major amputations

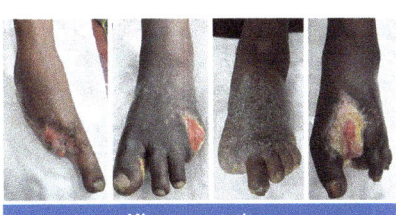

Minor amputations

Preventing Diabetic Foot Amputation

- Stratify people according to level of risk
- Not everybody with diabetes carry same risk of ulceration and amputation
- High risk patients are those who already have peripheral neuropathy, peripheral arterial disease, and previous history of ulceration or amputation
- Those at high risk need intensive education that involves practical demonstration
- Patients at high risk requires significant behavioral changes
- People need to learn to identify any problems that occur early
- Footwear is the most common cause of ulceration
- Problems should be identified early and treat promptly
- Health professionals need to be specially trained in caring people with diabetic foot disease.

Nonulcerative Pathology of Ulcers

These are the lesions, can be taken care to prevent an ulcer, amputation, and even death.

Callus formation

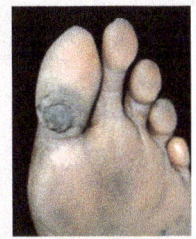
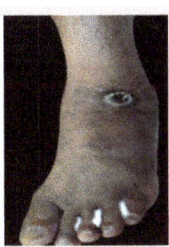

Fungal infection

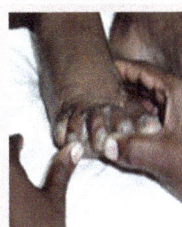
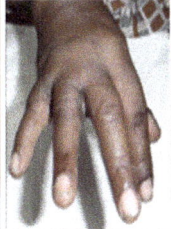

Dry skin, fissure, and cracks

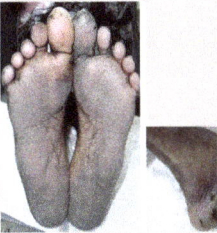

Contd...

Contd...

Deformity of nails, hypertrophy of the nail	
Herbal traditional marks	
Blisters	

Social Factors of the Diabetic Foot

- Social factors leading to diabetic foot ulcers are due to:
  - Bare foot walking
  - No proper foot wear
  - Poor hygiene of the foot
  - Lack of awareness among patients, relatives, friends, and health care workers
  - Poor living condition leading to rat bites, etc.
  - Tendency of patients to start home treatment
  - Visit to faith healer, herbal healer, etc.
  - Lack of facilities at primary health care, district or regional health care centers.

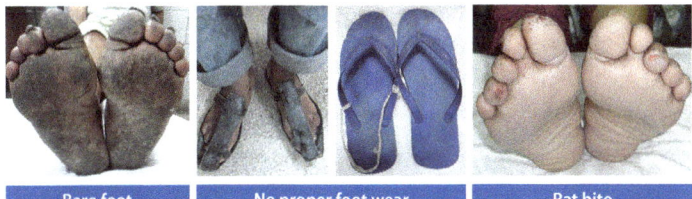

| Bare foot | No proper foot wear | Rat bite |

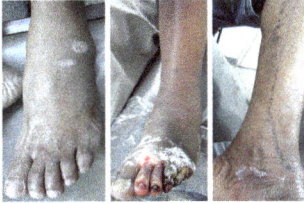 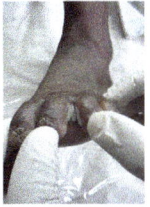 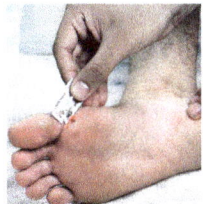

| Faith and herbal healer | Fungal infection | Home treatment |

Time is Tissue in the Diabetic Foot

- Typical sequential timeline of patients decision to seek help
  - Firstly, patient initiate treatment at home
  - Secondly, visit to faith or herbal healer
  - Thirdly, visit to primary health care center
  - Fourthly, visit to the district health care center
  - Fifthly, visit to regional health care center
  - By the time patient is referred to hospital it is often too late to save foot or prevent death.

Time is not tissue—these feet have history of weeks/months of ulcer, inability to walk, infection, misdiagnosis, and treatment.

Time is tissue—early reorganization and treatment of diabetic foot could avoid minor and/or major amputation even death of the patient.

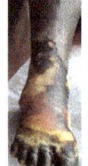 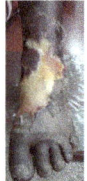 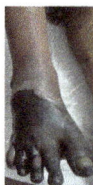 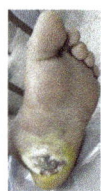 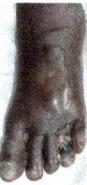 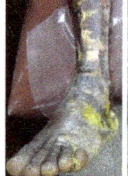 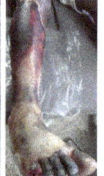

Late presentation

Pathway to Clinical Care for Diabetic Foot Ulcer

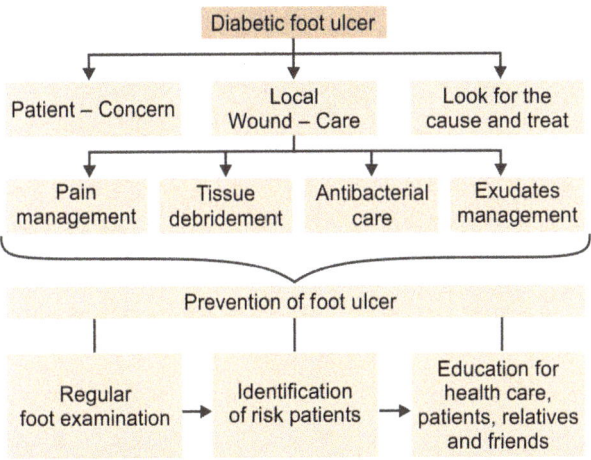

Risk Categorization System

Category	Risk profile	Check-up frequency
0	No sensory neuropathy	Once a year
1	Sensory neuropathy	Once every 6 months
2	Sensory neuropathy and signs of Peripheral vascular disease and/or foot deformities	Once every 3 months
3	Previous ulcer	Once every 1–3 months

How to Prevent Foot Problems

- Foot examination should be performed in patients with diabetes at least once a year and more frequently in those patients at high risk of foot ulceration
- Identification of patients at risk of ulceration is the most important aspects of amputation prevention
- Education, an integral part of prevention, should be simple and repetitive
- Education should be targeted at both, patients, family, relatives, friends, and health cares
- Appropriate foot wear is important
- Treatment of nonulcerative pathology–action should be taken.

Ulcer Prevention

Casting
- Nonremovable total contact casting or walker boot can be effective and safe for weight bearing treatment to prevent ulcers in Charcot's neuro-osteoarthropathy.

Footwear
- Therapeutic foot wear found to have significant lower incidence of foot ulcer.

Surgical Offloading
- Achilles tendon lengthening
- Single or pan-metatarsal head resection
- Joint arthroplasty
- Osteotomy
- Digital flexor tendon
- Other procedures like flexor hallucis longus tendon transfer, plantar fascia release, or Achilles tenotomy.

Training of Health Care Workers

The Step-by-Step Diabetic Foot Project

- The Step-by-Step training program is an organized focused course on diabetic foot
- Creating awareness of diabetic foot problems
- Reducing the risk of lower limb complications in people with diabetes
- Empower people with diabetes to care for feet
- Detect problems early and seek timely help when problem arise
- Providing sustainable training of healthcare professionals in diabetic foot
- Facilitating the transfer of information and expertise among health care workers
- Export ideas to other developing countries
- The potential benefits of the Step-by-Step Diabetic Foot program particular for less developed countries, is to manage the diabetic foot with limited human and financial resources more effective.

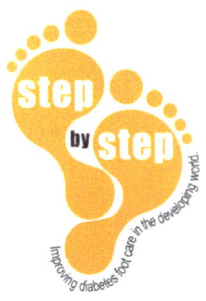

The Step-by-Step Diabetic Foot Project

- Birth of the Step-by-Step Foot project took place in Dar es Salaam, Tanzania, in 2003
- Pilot project conducted in Tanzania and India in 2004
- Update 8 courses of step by step have been conducted in Tanzania
- Two projects were for surgeons for the first time only in Tanzania
- Step-by-Step conducted in twelve countries in African continent
- Later it was exported to Asia, Middle East, Caribbean, and Europe
- This is the only project started from developing world—Tanzania and exported to other developing countries and now to developed countries
- Step by step leads to Train the Trainer Program.

The Step-by-Step Diabetic Foot Project in Tanzania

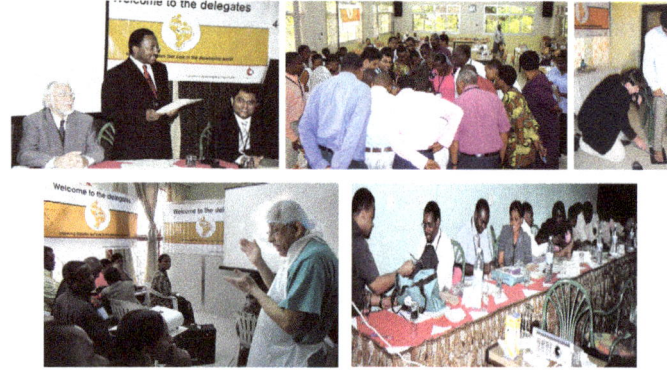

Train the Foot Trainer Project

- Step by step leads to formation of the Train the Foot Trainer (TtFT) program which has now being successfully executed in four regions across the globe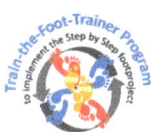
- First TtFT program was done in December 2012 for South America was successfully conducted in Brazil, participants from 14 countries of the South and Central America (SACA) region participated in the course
- This followed by Caribbean Island 22 countries, in Europe 17 countries and this year TtFT program was conducted for Western Pacific in Bangkok, Thailand
- In future Step-by-Step Diabetic Foot project will be going to Africa, Asia, and North America.

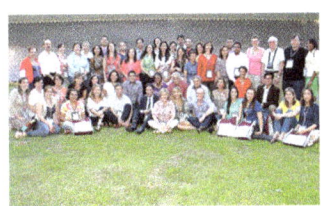
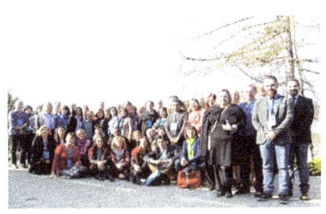
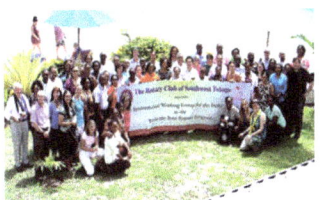
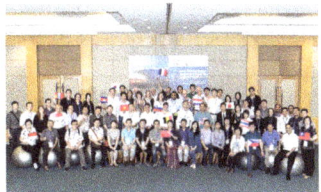

Organization of Foot Care

- Effective organization requires systems and guidelines for education, screening, risk reduction, treatment, and auditing
- There is strong evidence that the institution of a multidisciplinary foot-care team reduces amputation rates
- The specialist foot-care team must not only treat patients, but must also work in the primary care setting
- Make each patient a respected member of the team—you cannot succeed without their help.

The Minimal Foot Clinic Model

- Foot examination and detection of foot problems, such us callus, corns, nail pathologies, small wound, and infection
- Screening of the diabetic foot at risk
- Education on self-care of ulcers and infection
- Treatment of foot problems
- Preventive care with emphasis on education in foot care, foot wear, and trauma prevention.

Global New Concept

- First two boxes can be taken care at the lower level primary health care center or district health center
- Once an ulcer has to go to intermediate level district or regional health center
- Infection has to go to higher referral center.

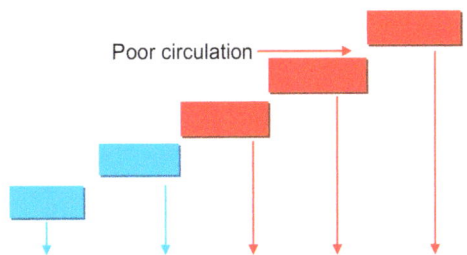

Pathway of Refer for Foot Care

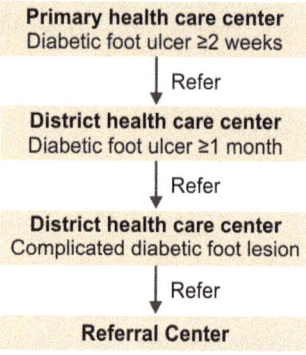

Tropical Diabetic Hand Syndrome

- Tropical diabetic hand syndrome is a complication affecting patients with diabetes in the tropics
- Syndrome encompasses a localized cellulitis swelling and ulceration of the hand to progressive, fulminant hand sepsis and gangrene affecting the entire limb
- Tropical; diabetic hand syndrome is less well recognized than foot infection and not generally classified as specific diabetic complication
- There is often history of minor hand trauma
- Presentation at the hospital is often delayed due to patient is not aware of potential risks, lack of concern, because the initiating trauma might have trivial, or decision to seek initial help form traditional healers
- Independent risk factors include poorly controlled diabetes, neuropathy, insulin treatment, or malnutrition.

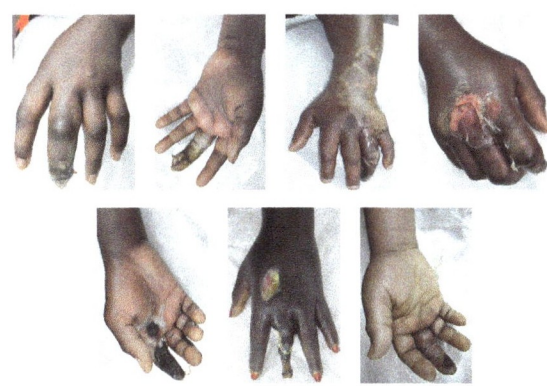

Algorithm for Management of Tropical Diabetic Hand Syndrome

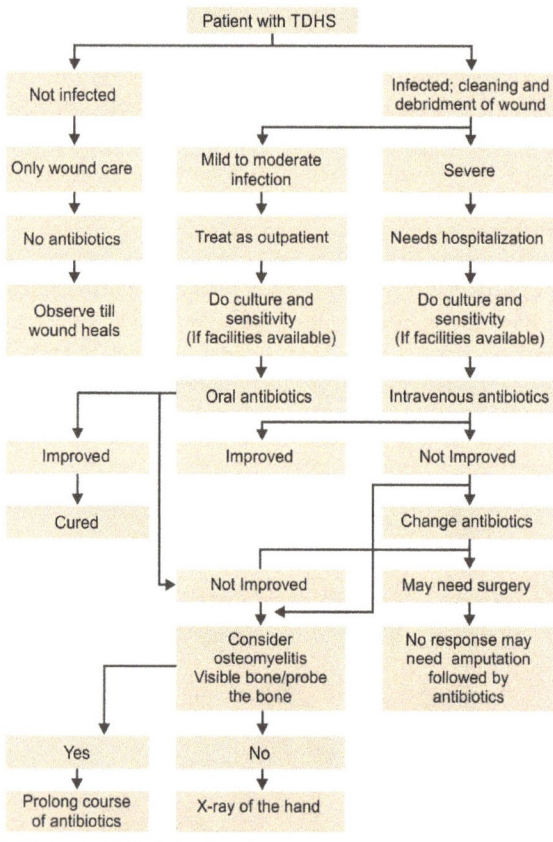

TDHS, tropical diabetic hand syndrome.

Issues—Particular Importance in Developing Countries

- These pocket guidelines must, of course, be adapted to the local circumstances
- Many aspects of the management of diabetic foot infections may differ from one developing country to other
- Physicians in developing countries may also face added difficulties
- They may not have access to a microbiology laboratory
- Antibiotic prescription, indigent patients may be unable to purchase the full course of therapy or may be prescribed inexpensive but potentially more toxic or less effective agents
- Home or work circumstances may make it very difficult for them to stay off their foot
- Affordability or be able to use an off-loading device
- May have traveled a long distance to see a physician and cannot easily return for follow-up visits
- Improving management of diabetic foot infections in developing countries will likely require a combination of education (for patients, pharmacists, and healthcare providers) and funding (for diagnostic, therapeutic, and preventative services).

Section 2

Surgical Aspect of Diabetic Foot

Diabetes Mellitus—Surgical Challenge

- Worldwide, diabetic foot ulcers and infection is a major public health problem
- More so in developing countries
- We need to understand that diabetic foot ulcer and infection is not primarily a surgical disease but complication/sequel of long standing metabolic derangement/disorder
- Therefore, we need team approach in the management of diabetic foot.

Team Approach

Minimum Members of the Team

- Diabetologist/endocrinologist/physician
- Surgeon
- Paramedic/diabetes educator.

Extended Team Can Include

- Dietician
- Wound care nurses
- Orthopedic surgeon
- Radiologist
- Infectious disease specialist
- Counselor
- Vascular specialist
- Nephrologist
- Cardiologist
- Physiotherapist.

Most important member of the team is patient and his family.

Foot Salvage Surgery

- Foot salvage surgery has to be done after proper assessment of patient's general and foot condition
- It is mandatory that prior to every foot surgery vascular assessment by means of ankle/brachial index by hand held Doppler
- Foot salvage surgery in diabetes is to be done on anatomical principal
- The concept of foot spaced needs to keep in mind
- Sub facial spaces and rigid spaces
- Three paces—medial, central, and lateral
- Toes cover these spaces like caps.

Neuropathy and Surgery

- Human foot is a very biomechanical structure and works with marvellous coordination
- However this balance is lost when it is affected by neuropathy
- Foot examination involves assessing extent of limited joint mobility, Intrinsic muscle strength, and toes deformities
- Crowding of toes in the presence of sensory neuropathy causes web space fungal infection which is important cause of foot abscesses in developing countries
- Tibialis anterior tendon also overacts inverting the foot causing increased pressure on lateral side of the foot and resulting in ulceration
- Tibialis anterior and Achilles tendon overact leading to plantar flexion and eversion of foot increasing pressure on forefoot and lateral side of foot resulting in ulceration
- Both these problems can be overcome by correcting balance of the foot by subcutaneous tendo-Achilles lengthening and transfer of tibialis anterior tendon.

Charcot Foot

- It is usually under diagnosed
- Usually unilateral edema in diabetes patients with neuropathy with warmth is treated as cellulitis
- Usually triggered by minor trauma in the presence of neuropathy/ ephropathy and retinopathy
- Patient continues his activity in the due to loss of protective pain sensation
- Minor trauma further increases blood supply triggering osteoclastic activity
- Ongoing trauma due to weight bearing walking, poor glycemic control, peripheral neuropathy causes destruction of ligaments and joint capsules leading to destruction of foot
- Early diagnosis, aggressive conservative treatment can prevent further irreparable damage to the foot.

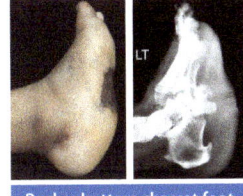

Rocker bottom charcot foot

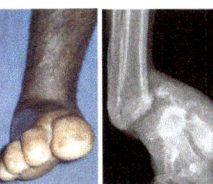

Charcot foot ankle dislocation pre- and postoperative

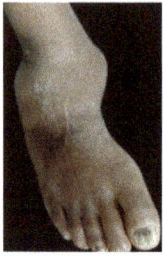
Charcot foot dislocation preoperative

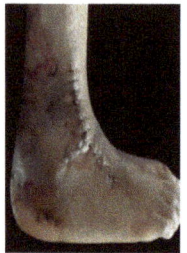
Postoperative after surgical correction

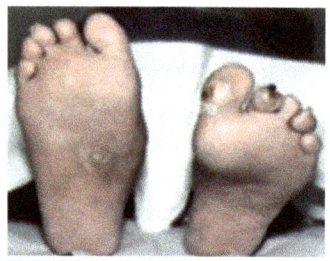
Bilateral Charcot foot deformities

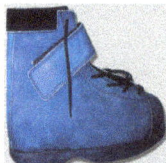
Shoes for healed Charcot foot with stabilization

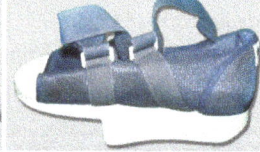
Front wedge sandals forefoot ankle wound off loading

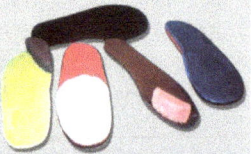
Toe and partial foot fillers

Imaging in Charcot Foot

Plain Radiographs

- Help to stage disease
- Help to determine if active disease is present or if the joint is stable (monitor serial radiographs)
- Help to identify osteopenia, periarticular fragmentation of bone, subluxations, dislocations, fractures, and generalized destruction.

Bone Scan (Not Always Ordered)

- A bone scan helps to differentiate between Charcot arthropathy and osteomyelitis
- An indium-111 white blood cell (WBC) scan often is used because it is more specific than the technetium-99m scan
- The WBC scan is a triple-phase bone scan that is often used to help confirm the diagnosis of osteomyelitis (positive in all phases).

Magnetic Resonance Imaging

- Allows for anatomic imaging of the area
- May help to distinguish between osteomyelitis and Charcot arthropathy.

Doppler Ultrasound

- It is used to rule out deep vein thrombosis
- It can be used in cases with peripheral artery disease.

Indication for Surgical Treatment

- Failure of conservative treatment
- Recurrent ulcerations
- Unstable foot
- Bilateral disease
- Obesity
- Higher activity level
- Younger age group.

Surgical Treatment for Charcot Foot

- Surgical procedures and techniques based on the location of the disease and on surgeon preference and experience with Charcot arthropathy
- Surgical procedures include:
  - Exostectomy of bony prominence
  - Osteotomy
  - Arthrodesis
  - Screw and plate fixation
  - Open reduction and internal fixation
  - Reconstructive surgery
  - Fusion with Achilles tendon lengthening
  - Autologous bone grafting
  - Amputation.

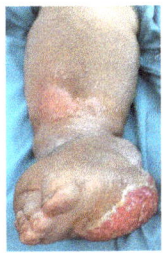
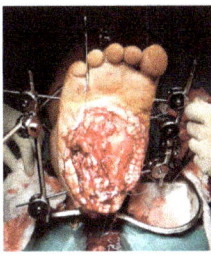

Charcot foot with mid and hind foot dislocation and infected large wound

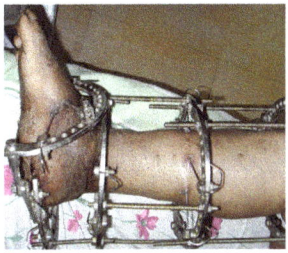

Charcot foot surgical correction with Ilizarov`s technique

Choice of Surgical Procedures

- Surgical methods can be based on Schön's classification system
- Open reduction and internal fixation should be used for an ankle with displaced fractures
- Ankle arthrodesis is necessary in patients with tibiotalar destruction
- In cases in which the hind foot has avascular necrosis of the talus, a talectomy with tibiocalcaneal fusion is necessary
- Arthrodesis may be necessary for patients with hind foot involvement
- For a mid foot pattern, surgical correction of rocker-bottom deformity and osteotomies for bony prominences are used
- If there is an associated hind foot/ankle equinus contracture, then a posterior release/Achilles tendon lengthening procedure is required
- For forefoot patterns, patients with bony prominences or recurrent ulcerations may need a resection arthroplasty.

Healing Time in Surgical Treatment of Charcot Foot

- Ankle: Mean time, 83 days, ± 22 days
- Hind foot: Mean time, 97 days, ± 16 days
- Mid foot: Mean time, 96 days, ± 11 days
- Fore foot: Mean time, 55 days, ± 17 days.

Complication of Surgical Treatment

- Soft tissue infection
- Deep vein thrombosis
- Problems with implants
- Failure of fusion
- Osteomyelitis
- Overall success rate of 75–80%.

Peripheral Arterial Disease and Surgery

- Fifteen percent of diabetes patients get peripheral arterial disease
- Usually ischemia is secondary to neuropathy
- Arteries affected are usually infrapopliteal vessels in majority of patients
- Below knee posterior tibial arteries is mainly affected
- Peripheral arterial disease in diabetes can be largely prevented by regular annual vascular assessment
- If on annual examination ankle-brachial pressure index is declining then Doppler should be done to assess formation of atherosclerotic plaques
- At this stage medication can help in development of good collateral circulation.

How Peripheral Arterial Disease is Different in Diabetes than Nondiabetic Patients

- Walking does not improve perfusion pre- and post-treatment in diabetic patients with wounds
- Claudications may be late presentation or may be absent
- Diabetic patient with severe ischemia may not get rest pain till there is impending gangrene
- Palpable pulses is not always a sign of optimal perfusion
- Postoperative off loading of the affected foot till wound heals is mandatory
- Toe pressure and transcutaneous oxygen concentration are the gold standards.

Peripheral Arterial Disease, Transcutaneous Oxygen Pressure, and Surgery

- Diabetic patients usually do not get claudication as they have sensory neuropathy
- It also must be understood that palpable pulse is not real indicator of good vascular supply as the distal pulses are usually fed by collateral circulation
- Gold standard for assessing vascular supply is measurement of transcutaneous oxygen pressure (TcPO$_2$) and toes pressure
- TcPO$_2$ is usually 40 mm or above
- If it is between 20 and 40 mm then chance of wound healing is moderate
- If it is below 20 mm then wounds are unlikely to heal
- Toe pressure is usually 40 mm.

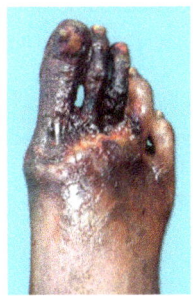 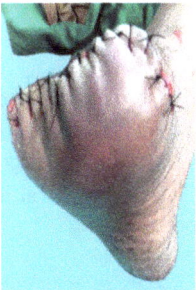

Forefoot gangrene after revascularization and after forefoot amputation

Imaging Modalities

- Every patient of peripheral arterial disease with wound when ankle-brachial pressure index is low or transcutaneous oxygen pressure is below 20 should be subjected to suitable for imaging for assessment of vascular supply to decide about type and feasibility of revascularization
- Patient with nephropathy who have albuminuria, glomerular filtration rate of less than 40 or serum creatinine of more than 1.5 mg need special consideration
- Pre-imaging protocol is as follows:
  - Check cardiac function
  - Patients with low left ventricle ejection fraction (LVEF) are high risk
  - Stop metformin
  - Start acetylcysteine 48 hours before angiography
  - Unless there is specific contraindication like very low LVEF patient should be well hydrated
  - Estimation of renal function tests
  - Patient who are already on dialysis of any type should undergo dialysis pre- and post-angiography
  - If patient is in sepsis local limited debridement to control the sepsis prior to imaging.

Selection of Type of Imaging

- Most useful and appropriate modality of imaging is digital subtraction angiography (DSA)
- This form of angiography gives useful information to take decision about revascularization
- If endovascular revascularization is feasible then it can be done at the same time
- Digital subtraction angiography cannot be done when patient's renal profile is deranged as the dye can cause further renal derangement
- In elderly (above age of 70 years) patients magnetic resonance angiography is preferable to assess feasibility of revascularization
- Computed tomography angiography is a good modality in patients who have chronic insufficiency
- However, main drawback is calcification of vessels can give false positive findings
- Patients who have acute problems like impending gangrene, severe foot infection and who are on some form of dialysis should be subjected to DSA as quick revascularization is required.

When and How to Treat Foot Gangrene When Revascularization is not Feasible

- Every patient of foot gangrene who cannot be subjected to revascularization does not need higher level amputation
- When rest pain is absent
- When there is no evidence of infection
- When lesion is limited to toes or part of toes
- When patient is metabolically and hemodynamically stable.

Selection of Type of Revascularization

- Majority of lesions can now with advances in technology can be revascularized with endovascular therapy
- Stenosis and blocks even up to length of 15 cm can be corrected to endovascular therapy
- Eighty percent of peripheral arterial disease can be corrected with endovascular therapy
- Multiple areas of stenosis/blocks may require hybrid therapy consisting of angioplasty and bypass graft
- Longer segment blocks in proximal vessels (aortolliac) with infrapopliteal stenosis may be corrected with hybrid therapy
- long stenosis in the range of 12–18 cm usually require bypass grafts.

Steps to Prevent Acute Kidney Injury in a Susceptible Patient

Preprocedure

- Fluids: Normal saline drip with bicarbonate started 12 hours before the administration of contrast and continued for 12 hours post-procedure
- N-Acetyl cysteine (NAC): 1200 mg intravenous/oral twice a day started 2 days before and continued 2 dated after.

Intraprocedure

- Minimum use of contrast
- More dilution to decrease volume
- Iodixanol- nonionic dimer, equal osmolarity as plasma.

Postprocedure

- Continue hydration and NAC
- Monitor renal function and watch the trend
- Very rare need for dialysis.

Use of Non-iodine Based Contrast

- Gadolinium can be used for borderline raised glomerular filtration rate
- Carbon dioxide (CO_2) impressive contrast medium with wide applications.

Carbon-dioxide Angiography

- Pressurized gas is injected through the catheter in large volumes
- Hospital grade CO_2 necessary
- Special high pressure syringe system used
- Gas injected in large amount at high pressure
- Displaces blood in the vessel
- Seen as a white in color versus contrast black
- Gas dissolved rapidly in blood—carried to lungs—excreted
- No upper safety limit for injection.

Advantages

- Decrease total volume of iodinated contrast
- Decrease total volume of fluid injected, important for angiography in children.

Disadvantages

- Increases cost
- Fragmentation in blood stream will yield poor images

- If enough volume is not injected—inadequate gas will reach the target site—under diagnosis of stenosis
- Poor visualization of smaller arteries
- Poor visualization in patients with poor breath hold.

Contraindications

- Severe right ventricular failure
- Known atrial septal defect/ventricular septal defect
- Chronic pulmonary obstructive disease or any other disease reducing lung capacity.

Post-revascularization Treatment

- Post-revascularization after 48 hours when patient is hemodynamically stable them proper debridement/local/minor amputation based on biomechanical principles should be done
- This can be done under regional anesthesia
- If revascularization is not optimal, $TcPO_2$ has not increased and only localized toe/toes dry gangrene is present then it is advisable to wait and continue conservative treatment
- If at the time of surgery vascular supply is adequate and all necrotic tissue has been removed partial or complete closure of the wound can be considered
- Adjunct therapy of hyperbaric oxygen/vacuum assisted closure therapy can be considered in patients whose wound shows necrosis or have suboptimal revascularization
- All patients postsurgery need culture specific antibiotics
- Strict glycemic, metabolic, and electrolyte management is essential.

Schedule for Antibiotics is as Follows

- If only soft tissue infection when complete removal of necrotic tissue is done: 2 weeks
- When infected bone is removed completely: 1–2 weeks
- If infected bone remains: 8–12 weeks
- Selection of antibiotics should be decided on following factors:
  - Comorbidities
  - Cost
  - Availability
  - Side effects
  - Tissue concentration
  - Minimum inhibitory concentration value
  - Route of administration and facilities/social support.

Post-revascularization Prevention

- All patients should have total offloading of affected foot/leg
- To prevent postoperative foot drop posterior plantar plaster support is essential
- After the wound heals gradual mobilization and skin care should be mandatory
- Proper footwear management should be done
- Recurrence can be avoided only by regular frequent follow up visits
- Patient education and training of relatives to take care is essential
- Many patients after prolonged illness and multiple procedures undergo depression
- Proper psychologically support is essential for wound healing and general recovery.

Necrotizing Fasciitis

- High incidence of necrotizing fasciitis (NF) in tropical countries with high humidity level patients with sensory, autonomic neuropathy are more prone
- Climate plays important part
- Autonomic neuropathy caused loss of sympathetic outflow causing shunts to open with gravity when patient starts his daily activity
- Neuropathy and hyperglycemia causes nonenzymatic glycation leading to changes in connective tissues and skin loosed its elasticity
- Cardinal clinical sign is proximally increasing subcutaneous induration
- Continuous activity in spite of increasing leg edema in the presence of advancing neuropathy causes microscopic breaks in epidermis giving portal of entry to bacteria
- This triggers inflammation which invades and causes necrosis of subcutaneous tissues and fascia
- If patient continues to walk weight bearing this necrosis rapidly spreads along the facial planes causing extensive destruction of tissues
- Another important cause, especially in Asian countries, is vigorous massage using counter irritant medicines to reduce swelling
- This causes separation and disruption of subcutaneous septae holding dermis to fascia and disrupting blood supply to dermis
- This leads to necrosis of subcutaneous tissue and fascia
- Necrotizing fasciitis which starts in foot or leg, unless treated aggressively in initial stages can rapidly spread to thigh and even to groin and abdomen due to anatomical fact that fascia in lower extremity is a continuous layer except at joint level where it is disrupted due to attachment to the joint
- Majority of the patients are severely ill and have multisystem affection
- Necrotizing fasciitis treatment needs to have very strong team approach

- For salvage necrotizing fasciitis peripheral arterial disease with peripheral arterial disease has very poor prognosis unless treated at early stage
- Revascularization in the presence of active sepsis is usually not possible
- Debridement has to be really extensive by removing all necrotic tissue keeping in mind preservation of anatomical integrity of the limb
- If fascia-septae dividing various compartments in leg and thigh are involved in necrosis then prognosis is usually poor
- This can be detected at early stage by magnetic resonance imaging
- In such cases early higher level amputation in necessary
- Necrotizing fasciitis usually is due to *Staphylococcus*
- If the treatment is delayed then infection becomes poly microbial
- Super added fungal infection occurs in patients who are further immune compromised with renal involvement
- Wound care in NF patients needs long term culture specific antibiotics, vacuum assisted closure-therapy, hyperbaric oxygen and reconstructive surgery to close the wound
- Necrotizing fasciitis usually has poor prognosis when pulmonary and renal involvement is present.

Necrotizing Fasciitis

Pre- and postoperative necrotizing fasciitis.

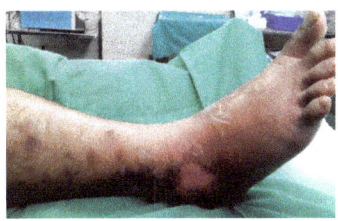

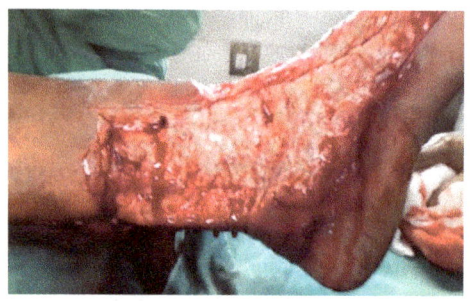
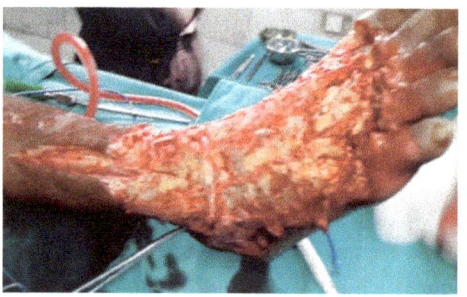
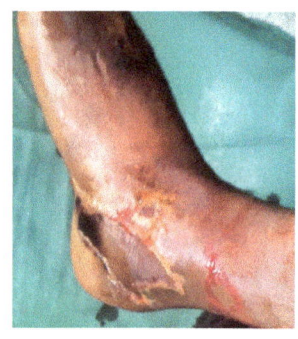
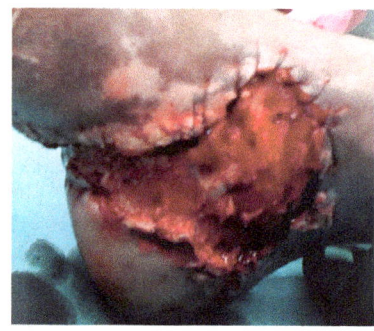

Necrotizing Fasciitis

Pre- and postoperative necrotizing fasciitis
Necrotizing fasciitis dorsum foot.

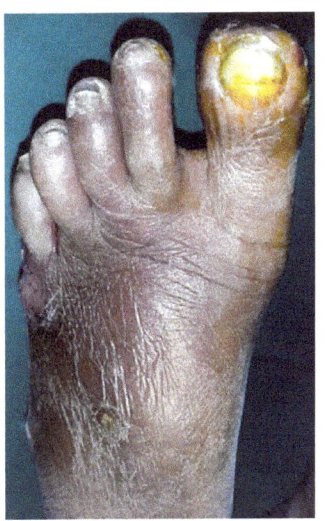
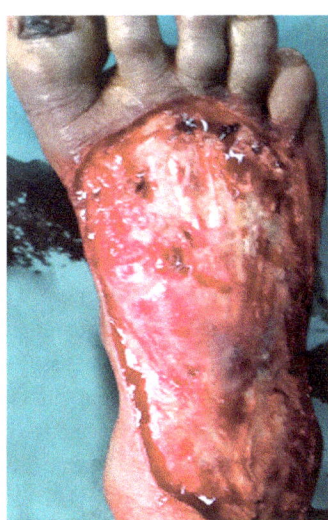

Osteomyelitis

- Commonest site of osteomyelitis is toes and/or metatarsal heads
- The commonest cause is bare foot walking in the presence of toe deformities and sensory neuropathy
- Hammer toe, mallet toe, claw toe are three commonest deformities
- Pressure ulcer on the tip of the toes can damage distal phalanx
- It is a myth that every patient osteomyelitis of toe needs amputation
- Meta-analysis of many studies have shown improved healing with conservative treatment
- If soft tissue infection is not severe then aggressive conservative treatment can help in saving the toe
- The conservative treatment of osteomyelitis includes:
  - Local debridement to remove necrotic tissue
  - Culture sensitivity of tissue sample
  - Culture specific antibiotics for 8–12 weeks
  - Off-loading of affected toe by foot wear modification
  - In case patient has nephropathy and culture report reveals multidrug-resistant organism with nephrotoxic antibiotics new technology of bio degradable culture specific antibiotic granules can be used for local delivery of antibiotics
  - In difficult to heal foot ulcers with osteomyelitis which do not heal even after all measures autologous growth factor concentrate can be used to inject locally to improve healing
  - Dressing with appropriate material
  - If the deformity is mobile the correction of toe deformity with flexor tenotomy
  - Strict glycemic control.

The Conservative Treatment of Osteomyelitis

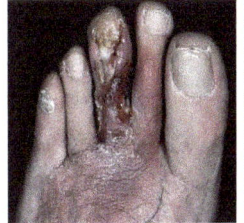
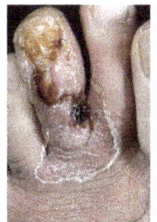
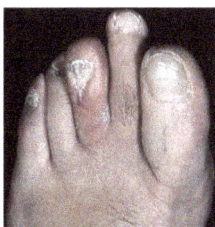

Osteomyelitis of third toe

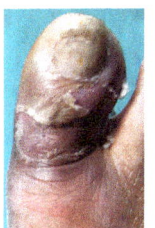
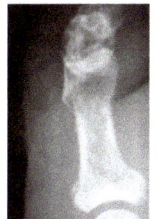
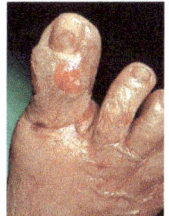
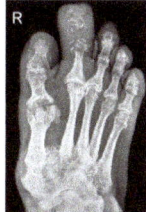

Osteomyelitis of big toe

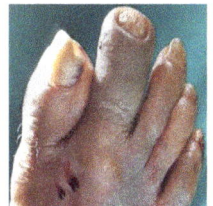

Osteomyelitis of second toe

Debridement in Patients with Infection and Vasculopathy

Preoperative Vascular Assessment Mandatory

- Local debridement before revascularization if wound is infected
- Total debridement after revascularization to reduce/removal necrotic load
- Total off loading till wound heals.

Postoperative Offloading is of Critical Importance

- All patients who have undergone foot surgery should have posterior plantar support to prevent foot drop
- Postoperative rehabilitation guidelines are as follows:
  - Gradual mobilization
  - Maturation of scar
  - Stretching of the scar
  - Foot exercise
  - Breaking in of the shoe
  - Extra care of contralateral foot.

Conservative Management of Localized Gangrene

- Total offloading of affected foot
- Low molecular weight heparin
- Anti-platelet drugs like cilostazol which improves collateral vascularity
- Dressing with povidone iodine to help in autoamputation
- Management of pain either by pharmacological therapy or paravertebral blocks
- Monitoring of metabolic, glycemic control
- Increasing pain denotes extension of necrosis
- Following dictum should be kept in mind—live tissue does not pain, dead tissue does not pain only dying tissue pains
- If patient becomes metabolically unstable and/or has unmanageable pain then higher level amputation is required.

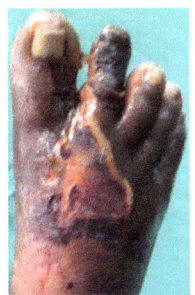 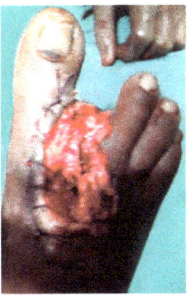

Necrotic toe infection with dorsal abscesses pre- and postoperative

Factors That Influence Wound Closure Procedure

Wound

- Location
- Depth
- Size
- Tissue extensibility/contracture
- Exudation
- Bacterial colonization.

Vascular

- Arterial insufficiency
- Venous insufficiency
- Lymphedema.

Deformity

- Charcot neuroarthropathy
- Underlying bone prominence
- Equinus.

Previous Infection

- Superficial (soft tissue)
- Deep (bone or joint involvement).

Host

- Controlled or uncontrolled diabetes
- Renal Insufficiency
- Coronary artery disease
- Congestive heart failure
- Anemia
- Hypertension
- Malnutrition
- Tobacco, alcohol, or drug dependency
- Ambulatory and functional status
- Age of the patient (life expectancy)
- Psychosocial
- Obesity
- Compliance.

Factors That Retard Healing

Local Factors

- Mechanical Injury
- Infection
- Edema
- Ischemia/necrotic tissue
- Topical agents
- Ionizing radiation
- Low oxygen tension
- Foreign bodies.

Regional Factors

- Arterial insufficiency
- Venous insufficiency
- Neuropathy.

Systemic Factor

- Inadequate perfusion
- Inflammation
- Nutrition
- Metabolic diseases
- Immunosuppression
- Connective tissue disorders
- Smoking.

Commonly Used Procedures within Each Surgical Category

Class	Description	Procedures	Potential risks for amputation
Class 1: Elective	Diabetic foot surgery procedures performed to treat a painful deformity in a patient without loss of protective sensation	<ul><li>Bunionectomy</li><li>Hammer toes repair</li><li>In-growing toenail removal</li><li>Metatarsal osteotomy</li></ul>	Very low
Class 2: Prophylactic	Diabetic foot surgery procedures performed to reduce risk of ulceration in person with loss of protective sensation but without open wound	<ul><li>Bunionectomy</li><li>Sesamoidectomy Hammer toe repair</li><li>Metatarsal osteotomy</li><li>Charcot exostectomy</li><li>Achilles tendon lengthening</li></ul>	Low
Class 3: Curative	Diabetic foot surgery procedures performed to assist in healing open wound	<ul><li>Metatarsal head resection, pan-metatarsal reaction</li><li>Keller arthroplasty</li><li>Metatarsal phalangeal or interphalangeal joint resection</li><li>Plantar midfoot exostectomy</li><li>Partial midfoot amputation, digital, ray, transmetatarsal amputation</li><li>Chopartis (it is mid foot amputation), syme, partial calcanectomy</li></ul>	Moderate
Class 4: Emergent	Diabetic foot surgery procedure performed to limit progression of acute infection	<ul><li>Incision and drainage</li><li>Amputation at appropriate level</li><li>Staged partial foot amputation</li><li>Major amputation</li></ul>	High

Class 1: Elective

Diabetic foot surgery procedures performed to treat a painful deformity in a patient without loss of protective sensation.

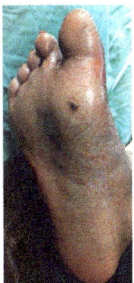
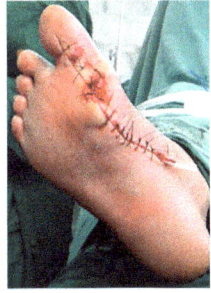

Tenosynovitis of flexor hallucis tendon

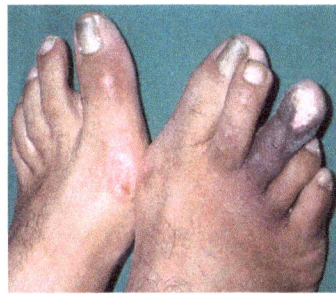

Toe deformities

Class 2: Prophylactic

Diabetic foot surgery procedures performed to reduce risk of ulceration in person with loss of protective sensation but without open wound.

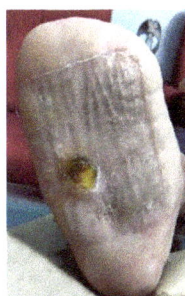

Post forefoot amputation causing midfoot callus due to biomechanical imbalance

Class 3: Curative

Diabetic foot surgery procedures performed to assist in healing open wound.

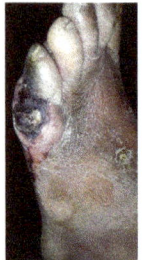
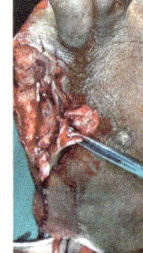

5th toe gangrene with 5th metatarsal ray excision postoperative

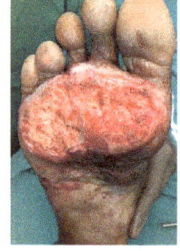
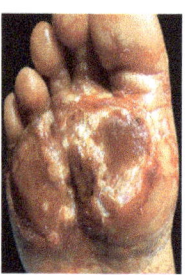

Thermal injury pre- and postoperative

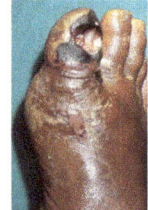
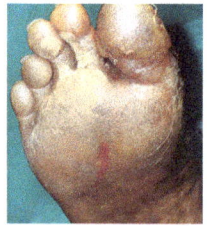
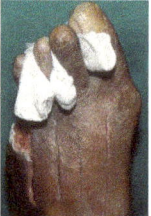

Web space fungal infection leading to toe necrosis/easiest way to separate toes to prevent fungal infection

Class 4: Emergent

Diabetic foot surgery procedure performed to limit progression of acute infection.

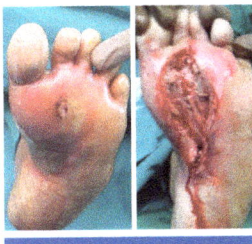

Infected callus 2nd metatarsophalangeal joint

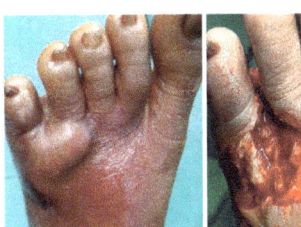

Web space fungal infection with abscess pre- and postoperative

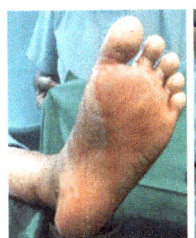

Abscess foot with flexor tendon infection pre- and postoperative

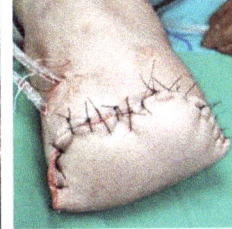

Below knee amputation

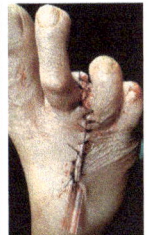

Metatarsal ray excision

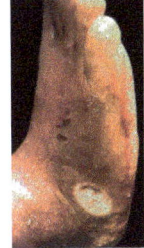

Infected dorsal ulcer causing osteomyelitis of mid tarsal

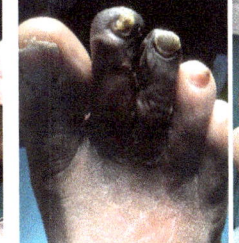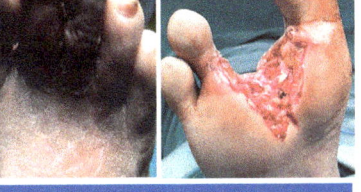

Toe gangrene pre- and postoperative

Different Types of Dressing

Dressing type	Indications
Impregnated guaze	Low exudates, granulating or epithelializing wound
Antimicrobials	Infected wounds
Enzymatic debridement	Slough necrotic wounds
Gels with silver	Mild to moderately exudating wounds with infection
Hydogels	Dry or necrotic wounds
Hydrocolloid	Low to moderate exudating wounds
Hydrocolloid with alginates	High exudating wounds
Aliginates	High exudates wounds
Foam	Moderate to high exudates
Foam with silver	Moderate to high exudates with infection
Hydrofiber foam	Moderate to high exudates
Hydrocapillary	Highly exudative wounds
Growth factors	Granulating wounds
Ionic silver	Infected wound
Hemostatic	Bleeding wound
Iodine with hyaluronic acid	Slough wounds
Collagen	Epithialzing wounds
Skin substitutes	Granulating epithialzing wounds

Acute Wound Flowchart

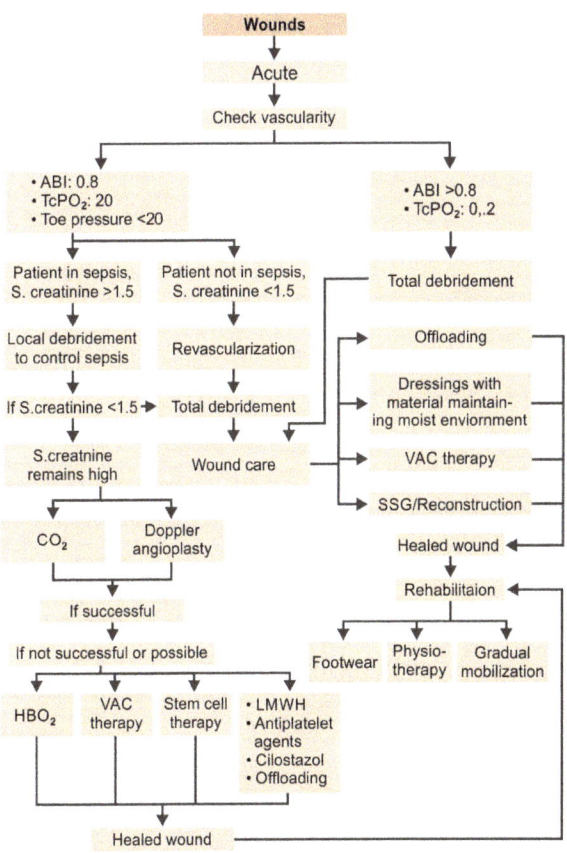

Chronic Wound Flowchart

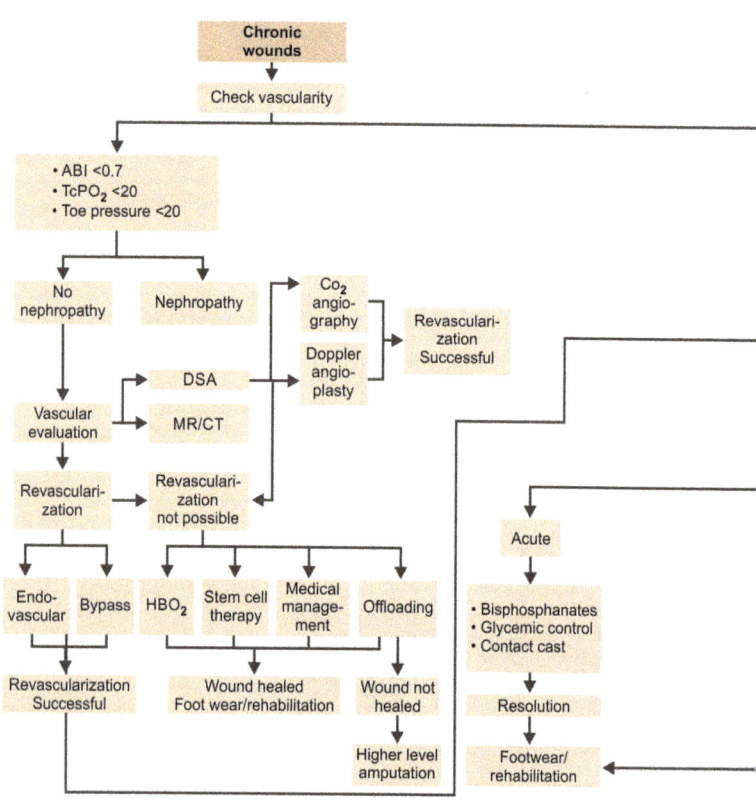

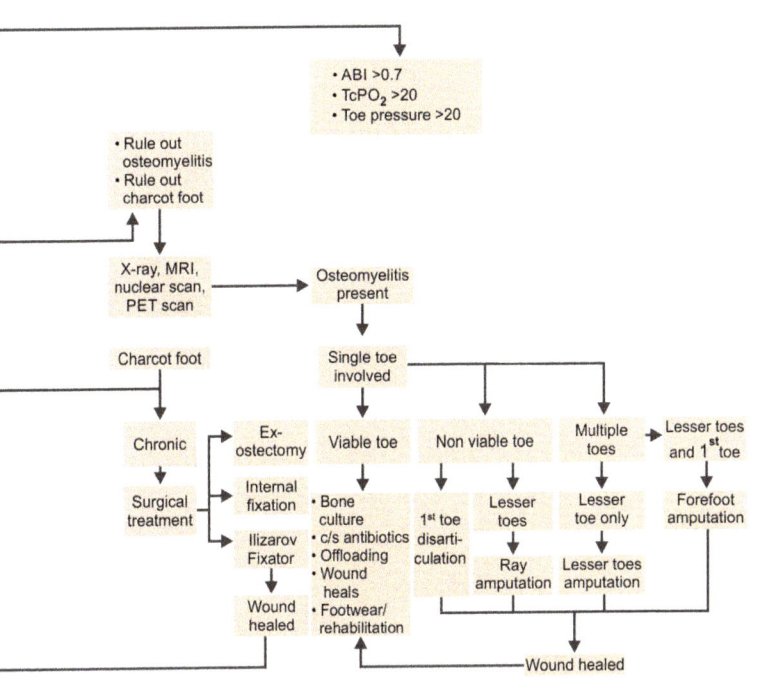

Skin Grafting in Diabetic Foot

Split Thickness Skin Graft

- Split thickness skin grafts offer many advantages in the management of diabetic foot wounds
- Graft can be applied to wounds
- With exposed healthy granulation tissue
  - Dermis
  - Fasicia
  - Muscles
  - Peritenon
  - Weight bearing areas.

Advantages of Split Thickness Skin Graft

- Easy take in the foot and lower extremity
- Better chance of survival in vascular compromised patients
- Reliable and minimally invasive
- Can cover large open wounds and amputations
- Cost effective if it needs to be repeated
- Useful for soft tissue defects on weight bearing areas
- Closing donors sites for local flaps or pedicle flaps.

Local Random Flaps

- Transport flaps
- Advancement flaps
- Rotation flaps.

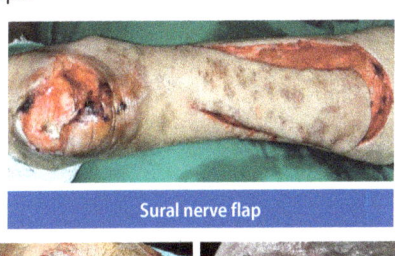

Sural nerve flap

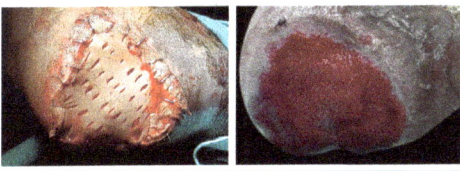

Heel wound pre- and post skin grafting

Axial Flaps

- Medial plantar artery flap
- Reverse sural artery flap
- Dorsalis pedis dorsal island flap.

Muscles Flaps

- Abductor hallucis flap for plantar and medial wounds
- Extensor digitorum brevis flap for small ankle defects, the lateral calcaneus, and lower tibial wounds
- Flexor digitorum brevis flap for plantar central wounds
- Abductor digiti minimi flap for tissue loss about the lateral aspects of the mid and rearfoot
- Surgeon often use this flap to close plantar lateral ulceration.

Free Tissue Transfer

- Radial forearm flap
- Rectus abdominal muscles flap
- Latissimus dorsi muscles flap.

Local/Regional Anesthesia for Diabetic Foot Surgery

Advantages of Local/Regional Anesthesia

- Can be used in seriously ill patients
- Does not need change in diet schedule
- Early control of septicemia
- Can be used repeatedly
- No postoperative nausea/vomiting
- No need of postoperative starving.

Lower Leg Block or Modified Ankle Block

- Deep peroneal nerve
- It can be blocked by injecting subcutaneously
- 3–5 mm along the lateral border of the shin with 2 mL of 2% xylocaine with 24G 1.5 inch needle.

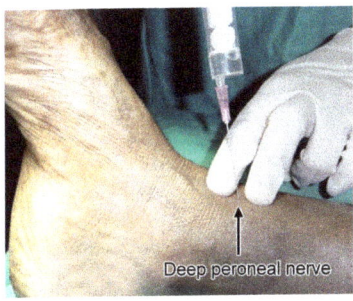

Lower Leg Block or Modified Ankle Block

- Posterior tibial nerve
- It can be blocked by injecting 3–5 mL of 2% xylocaine
- At the junction of proximal 1/3rd with distal 2/3rd of medial malleolus to calcaneum, where normally pulsations of posterior tibial artery is felt.

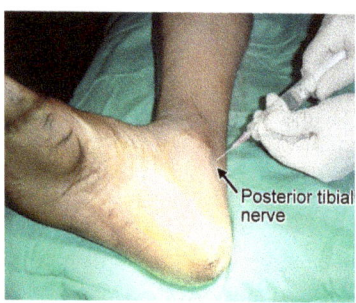

Lower Leg Block or Modified Ankle Block

- Sural nerve
- It can be blocked by injecting 2 mL of 2% xylocaine
- Between the tendo-Achilles and the calcaneum on the lateral aspect.

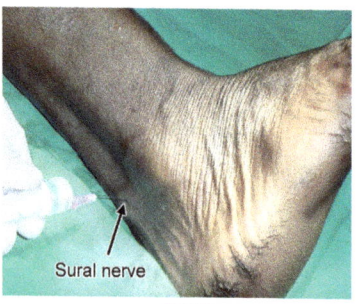

Lower Leg Block or Modified Ankle Block

- Ring block
- It can be blocked by injecting of 0.5% xylocaine
- Around the leg to block cutaneous nerves.

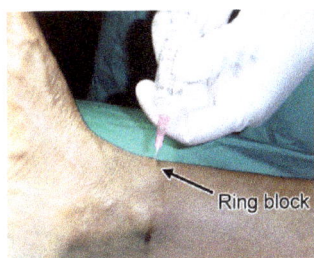

Mid Leg Block

- Anterior tibial nerve
- Inject 2–4 mL of 2% xylocaine subcutaneously 5–7 mm along the lateral border of the shin.

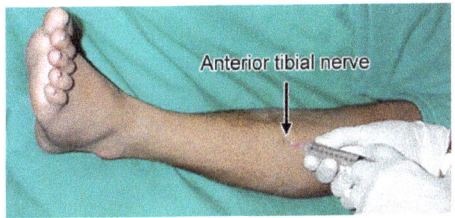

Mid Leg Block

- Posterior tibial nerve
- Spinal needle no 23G is inserted from the lateral side of the leg over the anterior border of fibula going medially downwards just to slip the interosseous border of tibia, advance 1–2 mm and deposit 8–10 mL of 2% xylocaine.

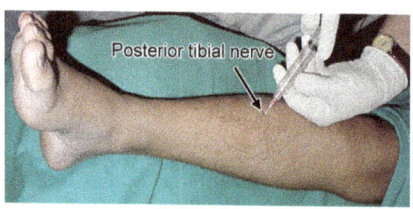

High Leg Block

- Anterior tibial nerve
- Inject 3–4 mL 2% of xylocaine 5–10 mm deep lateral to the upper end of shin.

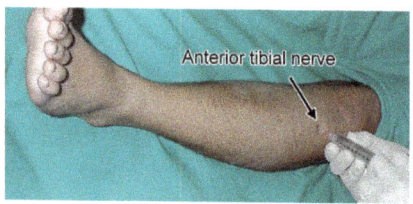

High Leg Block

- Posterior tibial nerve
- 2–4 cm below the neck of fibula – lateral approach spinal needle 23G is passed from lateral side of the leg over the anterior boarder of fibula going medially downwards just to slip the interosseous border of tibia, advance 1–2 mm and deposit 8–10 mL of 2% xylocaine.

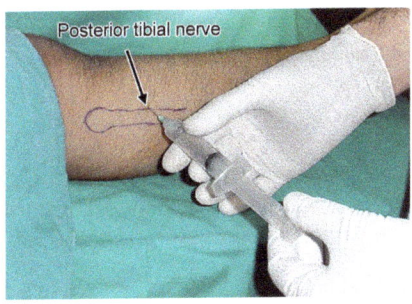

High Leg Block

- Lateral popliteal nerve
- 2–4 mL of 2% xylocaine injected around the neck of fibula

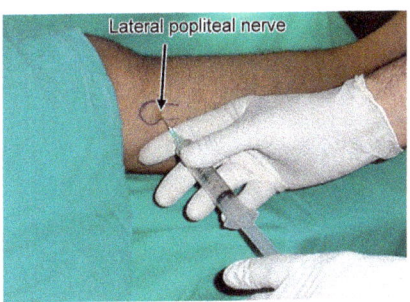

- An alternate technique if patient has a pain-free leg, then one may give sciatic nerve block in the lower third of thigh along with lateral popliteal nerve block and ring block.

Lower Leg Block or Modified Ankle Block

- Calcaneal nerve block
- Two finger breadth proximal to medial malleolus
- Inject along the direction of the nerve.

Mid Leg Block

- Sural nerve
- Inject 2–3 mL of 2% xylocaine along a line extended proximally tangential to the lateral border of the tendo Achilles.

Total Contact Cast for Diabetic Foot Patients

- Contact cast is gold standard of Charcot foot conservative treatment
- This needs to be applied for initial 2 weeks and then clinical and radiological review should be done at every follow up
- The cast needs to be continued till the affected foot temperature reduces.

Advantages of Contact Casting in Diabetic Foot Ulcers

- Maintains ambulation
- Reduces excessive plantar pressure
- Controls edema
- Protects foot from further damage
- Reduces the hospitalization.

Contraindication for Total Contact Casting in Diabetic Foot Ulcers

- Active Infection
- Ulcer depth greater than width
- Excessive leg swelling
- Uncontrolled diabetes
- Poor patient compliance.

Why Diabetes Patients Gets Bilateral Pedal Edema?

- Autonomic neuropathy causes loss of sympathetic out flow leading to dilatation arteriovenous shunts which diverts 30% blood by passing capillaries
- This coupled with nonenzymatic glycation makes skin less elastic causes edema
- Microscopic breaks in epidermis which is portal for entry for bacteria leading to necrotizing fasciitis
- Teaching patients to use deep vein thrombosis stockings can prevent this tragedy.

Wound Bed Preparation

- Dynamic and rapidly evolving concept
- Reduces the wound healing time
- Reduces the cost of the treatment
- Definition: Global management to accelerate endogenous healing and to facilitate other therapeutic measures
- It is third stage of wound care
- Earlier 2 stages are concept of moist wound healing and development of exogenous growth factors.

Evolution of Time Frame Work

- T = Tissue management
- I = Infection/inflammation control
- M = Moisture control
- E = Edge/epidermal/education control.

Tissue Management Debridement

- Removal of necrotic, devitalized, contaminated tissue
- Sharp and/or surgical debridement
- Necrotic tissue masks the infection
- Creates physical barrier to healing
- It inhibits constituents of extracellular matrix
- Prevents granulation tissue formation.

Selection of Types of Debridement

- Size, position, types of the wound
- Moisture level
- Pain management
- Time available
- Facilities available
- Level of health care training.

Types of Debridement

Surgical or Sharp Debridement

- Faster way to remove debris and necrotic tissue
- Minimal damage to the surrounding tissue
- Releases cytokines that helps wound repair
- Needs training
- Needs infrastructure.

Enzymatic Debridement

- Most selective
- Exogenous proteplytic enzymes are used to remove necrotic tissue
- Work with endogenous enzymes to degrade the necrotic tissue
- May cause minor transient pain and discomfort.

Enzyme Debridement

	Papain-urea	Collagenase
Debridement	+++	+++
Speed	++	+
Selective	-	+++
Pain	++	-
Maintenance debridement	-	++
Reduce bacterial burden	++	+++
Reduce exudates	++	++
More granulation tissue	++	-
Epithelization	-	++

Autolytic Debridement

- Natural debridement
- Phagocytic cells and proteolytic ezymes liquify and separate necrotic tissue
- Moist environment necessary for autolytic debridement
- Can result in to significant wound exudate
- Does not damage healthy tissue
- Requires minimal technology and training
- Minimal pain.

Biological Debridement

- Use of larvae/maggots
- Green bottle fly larvae
- Useful in patients with thick slough
- Limited availability
- Not accepted by many patients
- Eradicates infection and smell.

Mechanical Debridement

- Non selective method
- Wound irrigation, whirpool therapy, wet to dry dressing
- Significant discomfort and pain
- Wound irrigation is unsuitable for granulating wounds.

Maintenance Debridement

- An extended phase of debridement
- Required due to co morbidities
- Single episode of debridement may not be sufficient
- Offers distinct advantage in wound management
- Enzymatic and autolytic debridement is very useful.

Wound Bed Preparation

	Debridement	Optimal compression	Antiseptics	Dressings
Necrotic tissue	+++	+	++	+
Edema control	+	+++	+	+
Well vascular wound	++	+	+	+
Reduce bacterial burden	+++	++	+++	+
Minimize wound exudate	+	++	+++	+

Callus Debridement in Diabetic Foot

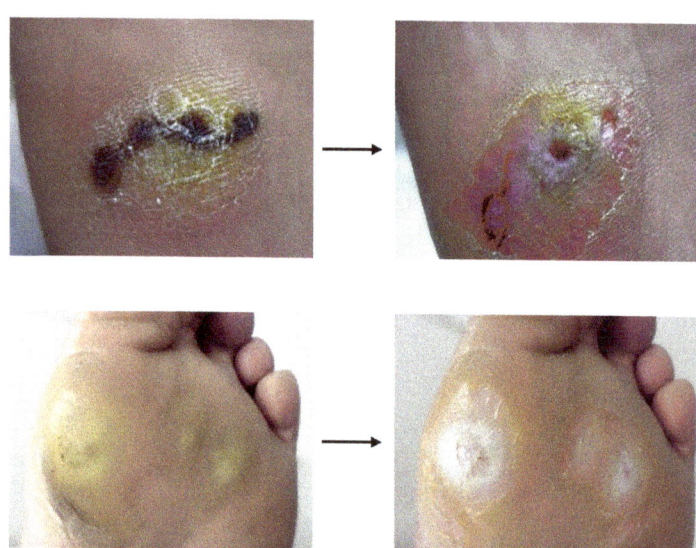

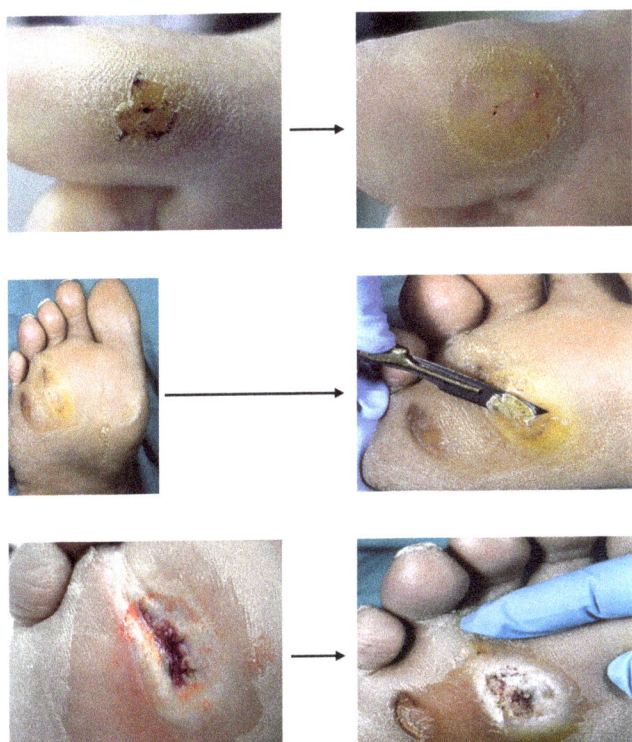

Adhesive Felt for Offloading

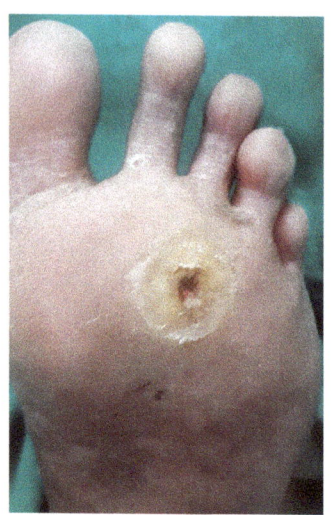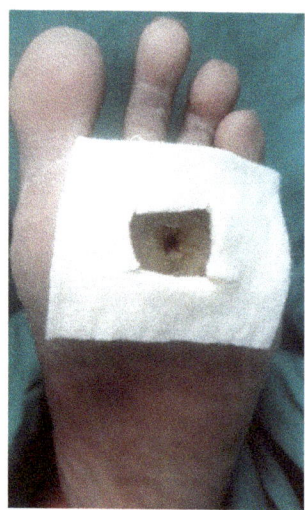

Pressure Relief Gel Pads and Support

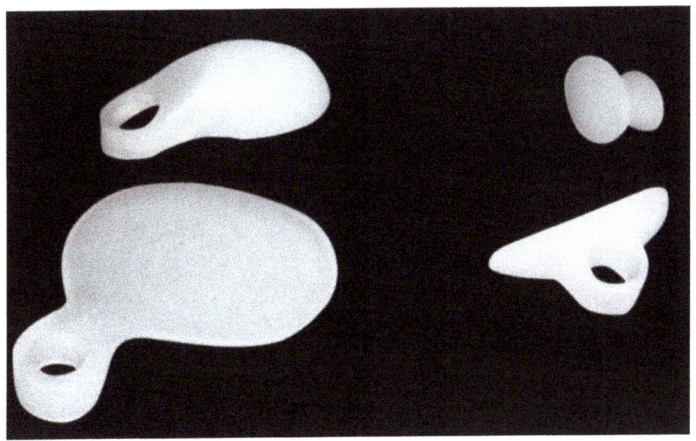

Deformed but Walkable Diabetic Feet

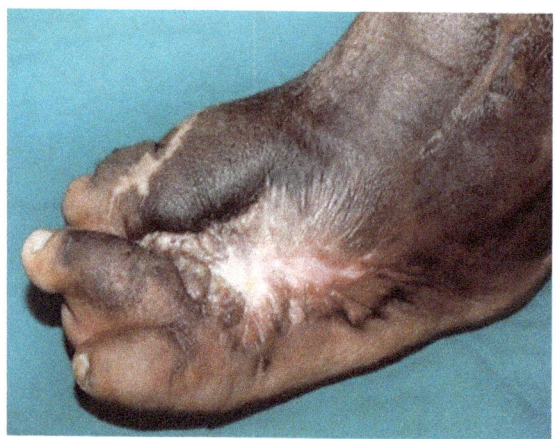

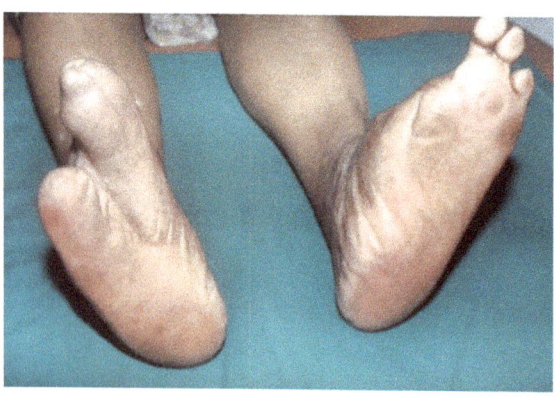

Vacuum-assisted Wound Closure

- Topical negative pressure therapy which can be used to achieve closure of diabetic foot wounds
- The pump applies subatmospheric pressure through a tube and foam sponge applied to the ulcer over a dressing and sealed in place with a plastic film
- The dressing is replaced every two to five days
- Small portable pumps are now available
- Negative pressure improves the dermal blood supply, and stimulates granulation which can form over bone and tendon. It reduces bacterial colonization and diminishes edema and interstitial fluid
- Vacuum-assisted closure therapy treatment is usually 10–15 days
- The effect may wear off after 3 days but if the pump is removed and then replaced after 1 day this restores the effect
- Excessive pain may prohibit the use of this technique (even in neuropathic feet).

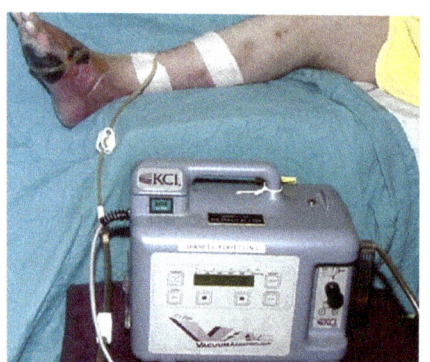
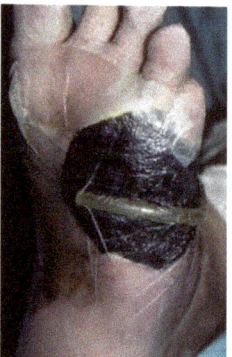
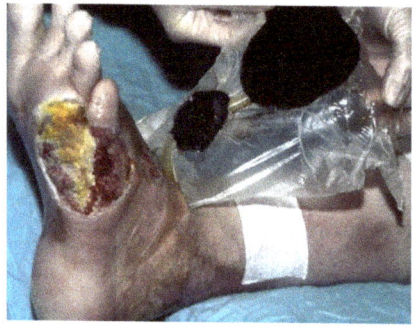

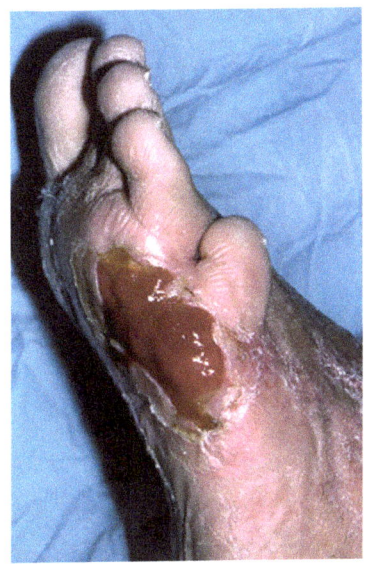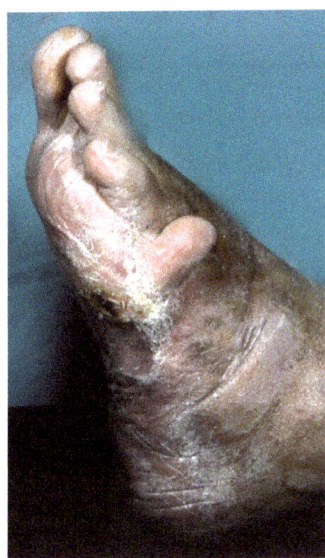

Footwear in Diabetes

Characteristics an Ideal Footwear in Diabetes

- Wide toe box
- Extra depth
- Appropriate insole
- Heel counter
- Rigid out sole
- Rocker adjustment to reduce the pressure.

Footwear Insole

Characteristics of an Ideal Insole

- 8–10 mm thick
- Shore hardness between 25 and 35
- Must distribute pressure equally over the fore foot
- Areas of stress isolation should be possible
- Should not bottom out
- Should protect high pressure area.

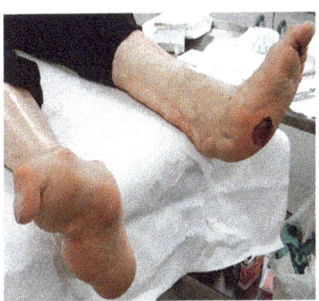
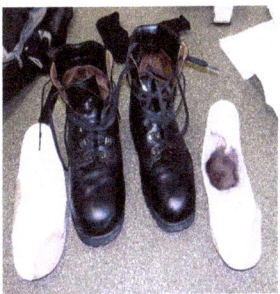

Moulded Insoles for deformed foot

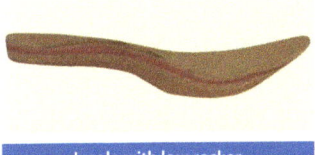

Insole with low rocker

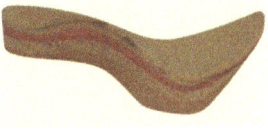

Insole with high rocker

Types of Insoles

- Microcellular rubber
- Closed cell foam
- Polyurethane foam
- Ethylene vinyl acetate
- Polymer
- Sorbothane
- Silicone gel.

Total Contact Orthosis

Objectives of total contact orthosis

- Relieve the areas of excessive plantar pressure
- Reduce the shock
- Reduce the shear
- Accommodate deformity
- Stabilize and support deformity
- Limit the motion of joints.

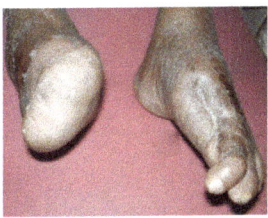
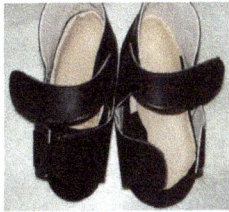

Footwear for bilateral deformed and partial foot

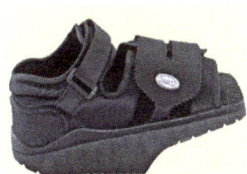
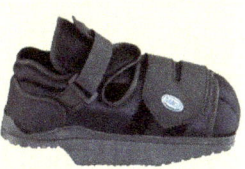

Offloading sandals

Rocker Outsole

Principles of Rocker Adjustment in Diabetic Footwear
- Minimize toe spring
- Maintain heel forefoot height difference
- Adjust the axis of rocker as per the individual patient
- Teach the patient not to take support of forefoot flat
- Flare out outsoles
- In shoe pressure measurement.

Pathology Causing Toe Injuries due to Deformities and Poor Foot Care/Footwear

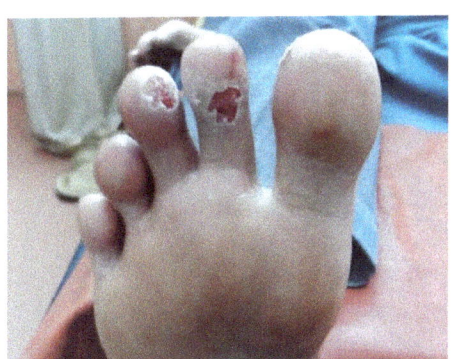
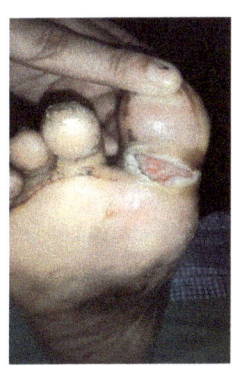
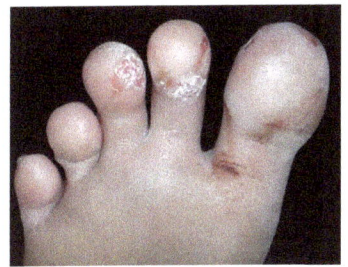
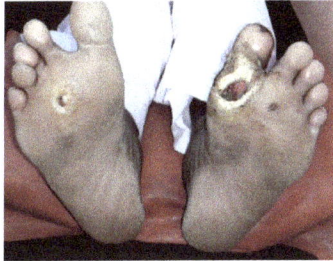

Guidelines for Footwear Prescription in Diabetes

Category 0: No Neuropathy

- Patient diagnosed with diabetes mellitus
- Protective sensation intact
- Ankle-brachial pressure index >0.8 and toe systolic pressure >45 mm Hg
- Foot deformity may be present
- No history of ulceration.

Possible Treatment

- Patient education
- Possible shoe accommodations
- Follow up 6–12 months.

Category 1: Neuropathy, No Deformity

- Protective sensation absent
- Ankle-brachial pressure index >0.8 and toe systolic pressure >45 mm Hg
- No history of ulceration
- No history of Charcot's joint.

Possible Treatment

- Same as category 0 plus
- Possible shoe gear accommodation (pedorthist/orthotist consultation)
- Quarterly visits to assess shoe gear and monitor for signs of irritation

- Follow up 3–4 months
- Patients are 1.7 times more likely to develop ulcer.

Category 2: Neuropathy, with Deformity

- Protective sensation absent
- Ankle-brachial index >0.8 and toe systolic pressure >45 mm Hg
- No history of ulceration
- No history of Charcot's arthropathy
- Foot Deformity present (focus of stress).

Possible Treatment

- Same as category 1 plus
- Pedorthist/orthotist consultation for possible custom—moulded/extra-depth shoe accommodation
- Possible prophylactic surgery to alleviate focus of stress
- Follow up 2–3 months
- Patients are 12.1 times more likely to develop ulcer.

Category 3: History of Pathology

- Protective sensation absent
- Ankle-brachial index >0.8 and toe systolic pressure >45 mm Hg
- History of neuropathic ulceration, amputation or Charcot's arthropathy
- Foot deformity present (focus of stress).

Possible Treatment

- Same as category 2 plus
- More frequent visits may be indicated for monitoring

- Follow up 1–2 months
- Patients are 36 times more likely to develop ulcer.

Category 4A: Neuropathic Wound

- All UT stage A wounds
- Protective sensation absent
- Ankle-brachial index >0.8 and toe systolic pressure >45 mm Hg
- Foot deformity normally present
- No acute diabetic Charcot's arthropathy.

Possible Treatment

- Same as category 3
- Pressure reduction program instituted
- Wound care program instituted.

Category 4B: Acute Charcot's Joint

- Protective sensation absent
- Ankle-brachial index >0.8 and toe systolic pressure >45 mm Hg
- Noninfected neuropathic ulceration
- Diabetic neuropathic osteoarthropathy (Charcot's joint present).

Possible Treatment

- Same as category 3
- Pressure reduction program instituted
- Thermometric and radiographic monitoring
- If ulcer is present, treatment is the same for category 4A.

Category 5: The Infected Diabetic Foot

- All UT stage B wounds
- Infected wound
- Charcot's arthropathy may be present.

Possible Treatment

- Debridement of infected, necrotic tissue, and/or bone as indicated
- Possible hospitalization, antibiotic treatment regimen
- Medical management
- Offloading/modified footwear.

Category 6: The Ischemic Limb

- Ankle-brachial index <0.8 and toe systolic pressure <45 mm Hg
- Pedal transcutaneous oxygen tension <40 mm Hg
- Ulceration may be present
- All UT stage C and D wounds.

Possible Treatment

- Vascular consult, possible revascularization
- If infection present, treatment same as for category 5
- Consultation concomitant with control of sepsis
- Standard diabetic footwear/modified or moulded footwear.

Why Early Detection and Treatment of Critical Limb Ischemia

- 15–20% of diabetic patients have peripheral artery disease
- 1% of peripheral artery disease population represent critical limb ischemia
- Critical limb ischemia represents a challenging disease state associated with considerable morbidity and mortality in addition to a large financial impact on the society
  - At 1 year
  - 25% mortality
  - 25% amputation
  - 50% amputation free survival.
- Therefore patients with critical limb ischemia are at exceptionally high risk for cardiovascular events and most eventually die of cardiac or cerebra-vascular event.

Fungal Infection in Diabetic Foot

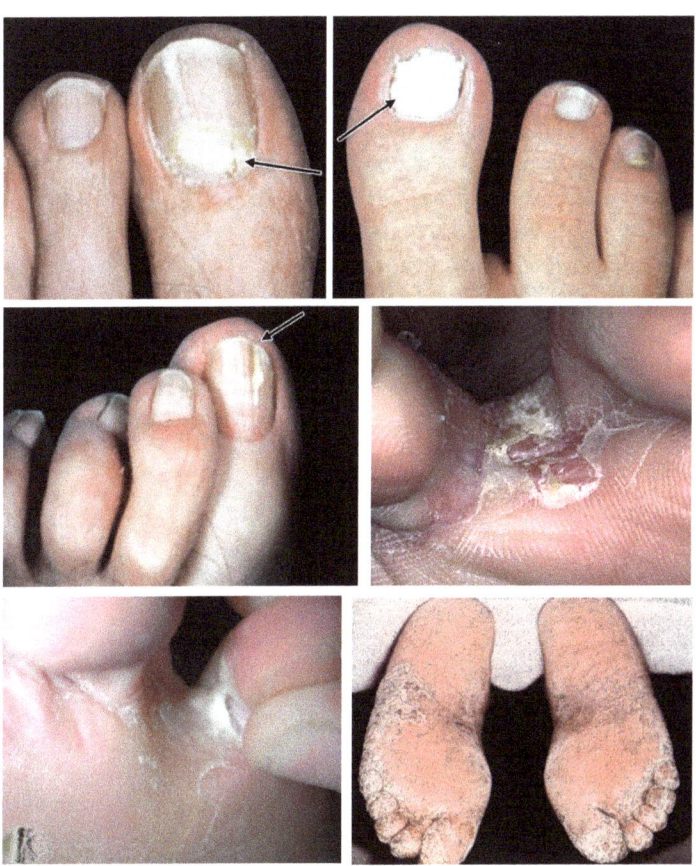

Ten Commandments of Foot Care in Diabetes

- Do not walk bare foot
- Inspect the feet daily for: Blisters, wounds, bleeding, hotness
- Do not apply hot fomentation/cold packs/strong ointments
- Use correct footwear
- Do not walk bearing weight on affected foot
- Do not sit crossed legged for long time
- Do not remove footwear during traveling
- Cutting nails regularly-trimmed square
- Do not cut corns/calluses with blades/knives set
- Clean the feet twice a day with soap and water and wipe web space dry and apply softening agent.

Wound Care Mini: Glossary

Diabetic foot	Infection, ulceration and/or destruction of deep tissues associated with neurological abnormalities and various degrees of peripheral vascular disease in the lower limb
Foot	The structure at or below the ankle
Foot lesion	Any abnormality associated with damage to the skin, nails, or deep tissues of the foot
High risk	Presence of or characteristics indicating high probability of developing a specific complication
Low risk	Absence of presence of few characteristics indicating a high probability of developing a specific complication
Healing	Intact skin, i.e., functional epithelialization
Necrosis	Devitalized tissue, either wet or dry, irrespective of tissue involved
Gangrene	A continuous necrosis of the skin an underlying structures (muscles, tendon, joint, or bone), indicating irreversible damage where healing cannot be anticipated without loss of some part of the extremity
Edema	Swelling of the foot sufficiently pronounced to leave a clear imprint of the pressure by a finger
Diabetic neuropathy	The presence of symptoms and/or signs of peripheral nerve dysfunction in people with diabetes, after exclusion of other causes
Neuroischemic	The combination of diabetic neuropathy and ischemia
Erythema	A pink or red discoloration that blanches to some degree on compression
Callus	Hyperkeratosis caused by excessive mechanical loading

Contd...

Contd...

Vascular	
Peripheral arterial disease	Presence of clinical signs such as the absence of the pedal pulses, a history of intermittent claudication, rest pain and/or abnormalities on noninvasive vascular assessment, indicating disturbed or impaired circulation
Critical limb ischemia	Persistent ischemic rest pain requiring regular analgesia for more than two weeks and / or ulceration or gangrene of the foot or toes, both associated with an ankle systolic pressure of <50 mm Hg or a toe systolic pressure of <30 mm Hg
Claudication	Pain in a foot, thigh or calf which is aggravated by walking and is relieved by rest, and is combined with evidence of peripheral vascular disease
Rest pain	Severe and persistent pain localized to the foot and frequently relieved by lowering the foot
Angioplasty	Re-establishment of an arterial lumen by percutaneous transluminal instrumentation/technique
Ulcer	
Superficial ulcer	Full thickness lesion of the skin extending through the subcutis, which may involve muscle, tendon, bone, and joint
Deep ulcer	Full thickness lesion of the skin extending through the subcutis, which may involve muscle, tendon, bone, and joint
Infection	
Cellulitis	Presence of swelling, erythema and heat. Indicating an inflammatory reaction, irrespective of cause
Infection	Invasion and multiplication of microorganisms in body tissues, which may be clinically inapparent or result in local cellular injury due to competitive metabolism, toxins, intracellular replication, or immune response

Contd...

Contd...

Superficial infection	An infection of the skin not extending through muscle, tendon, bone, or joint
Deep infection	Evidence of abscess, septic arthritis, osteomyelitis, or septic tenosynovitis
Osteitis	Infection of the bone without involvement of bone marrow
Osteomyelitis	Infection of the bone, with involvement of the bone marrow
Amputation	
Amputation	Resection of a terminal part of a limb
Primary amputation	The first amputation procedure in a sequence until a final outcome (healing or death)
First event amputation	The first primary amputation in an individual in a certain period, irrespective of side and level of amputation
Re-amputation	Amputation of an extremity with an unhealed previous amputation
New amputation	Amputation of an extremity with a healed previous amputation
Bilateral amputation	Simultaneous amputation of both lower extremities, irrespective of amputation level
Second leg amputation	Major amputation in a patient, who has had a previous amputation of the contralateral leg
Minor amputation	Midtarsal disarticulation or below
Major amputation	Every amputation above the midtarsal level
Amputation level	Toe disarticulation, ray amputation, transmetatarsal amputation, tarsometatarsal disarticulation, midtarsal disarticulation, ankle disarticulation, trans-tibial amputation (below knee), knee disarticulation (through knee), transfemoral amputation (above knee), and hip disarticulation

Contd...

Contd...

Miscellaneous	
Foot deformity	Structural abnormalities in the foot such as presence of hammertoes, claw-toes, hallux valgus, prominent metatarsal heads, status after neuro-osteoarthropathy, amputations, or other foot surgery
Debridement	Removal of dead tissue
Neuro-osteoarthropathy (Charcot-foot)	Noninfectious destruction of bone and joint associated with neuropathy
Non-weight bearing	Off-loading of a weight bearing area by the strict use of crutches, wheelchair, cast or other orthotic appliances
Therapeutic footwear	Footwear designed to relieve biomechanical stress on an ulcer and which can accommodate dressing
Protective footwear	Foot wear designed to prevent ulceration
Insole	The soft layer of the bottom of the inside of a shoe. Usually removable
Orthosis	An appliance which controls corrects or accommodates a structural or functional abnormality

Further Reading

1. Boulton AJM, Cavanagh PR, Rayman G. The Foot in Diabetes, Fourth edition, 2006.
2. Internationals Working Group on the Diabetic Foot (IWGDF). The development of global consensus guidelines on the management and prevention of the Diabetic Foot 2015. Available from: www.iwgdf.org.
3. Pendsey S, Contemporary Management of the Diabetic Foot, 1st edition 2014.
4. Preventive foot care programs. In: Hinchliffe R, Thompson M, Schaper N, et al., (eds.) The diabetic foot: Evidence based management. 1st edition. New Delhi: Jaypee Brothers Medical Publishers (P) Ltd.